The Good Grief Club

The Good Grief Club

A true story about the power of friendship and French toast

MONICA NOVAK

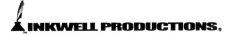
INKWELL PRODUCTIONS.

Cover design by Adam Mehlhaff
Cover photography by Kelly Axtolis

First Printing, January 2008

ISBN: 0-9766340-5-8
Library of Congress Control Number: 2001012345

Published by:
Inkwell Productions
10869 N. Scottsdale Road #103-128, Scottsdale, AZ 85254-5280
Tel: (480) 315-3781   Toll Free: (888) 324-BOOK (2665)
Email: info@inkwellproductions.com   Web: www.inkwellproductions.com

The author makes grateful acknowledgement for the following permissions:

Excerpt from *The Gift* by Danielle Steel (Delacorte Press, 1994) appears courtesy of Random House, Inc.

Centering Corp. for permission to quote from *Little Footprints: A Special Baby's Memory Book* by Dorothy Ferguson, Copyright 1989

NewSage Press for permission to quote from *Life Touches Life: A Mother's Story of Stillbirth and Healing* by Lorraine Ash, Copyright 2004

Perinatal Loss for permission to quote from *When Hello Means Goodbye* by Paul Kirk, MD and Pat Schwiebert, RN, Copyright 1981, 1985, 1993

UNITE, Inc. for permission to quote from "A Prayer for Spring" by Janis Heil, *UNITE Notes*, Spring 1984 issue, Copyright 1984 by UNITE, Inc., c/o Jeanes Hospital, 7600 Central Avenue, Philadelphia, PA 19111, (888) 48-UNITE

For Miranda, my precious baby, who has been with me every step of the journey. Your light shines on in my life.

Acknowledgments

The journey of writing this book began ten years ago when I was awakened in the middle of the night with an urgent sense that I should write down the details of this story. I didn't know then why it would be so important. One year later, while driving home from Indiana to Illinois, I came upon a late-night AM talk radio program being broadcast from Minnesota featuring author Barbara Glanz. As she talked about her own books, she encouraged people, like me, who had a story to tell but were mentally stuck because of a lack of formal writing education or experience. So first and foremost, I need to thank Barbara and my unseen "angels" for getting me on this road and keeping me behind the wheel with constant guidance and inspiration.

Thank you Pat Vaci, RN, Perinatal Support Services Coordinator at Advocate Good Samaritan Hospital in Downers Grove, Illinois, for your ceaseless compassion, support, and encouragement to me and Al during the months following Miranda's death, and in the years during the writing of this book. So many families have been blessed to have been led to you and the Share program at Good Sam.

Dr. Ross shared not only the most joyful moments of my life, but also the most painful. Thank you for being not just an extraordinary doctor, but for being a friend. Your compassion (and willingness to make house calls) is a shining example for all physicians, nurses, and the entire human race.

Candy Sibly, RN, sat with us during our earliest, most raw moments of pain with courage and compassion, guiding us gently through unspeakably difficult decisions, and for that we will be eternally grateful.

Thank you Rachel, Dawn, Heidi, Beth, Darlene, Wendy, and Tracy (in chronological order) and their husbands for sharing this journey with me and for sharing your stories with the world. This book wouldn't be what it is without your support, and I wouldn't be the person I am without your friendship and love.

To Kathy, whose courage to seek support and healing thirty years after her loss is an inspiration to me and to all who read her story. Thanks to you, and to Tim and Julie, for sharing your stories with me for the Prologue.

Thank you Lynne Schwartz for taking a chance and reaching out to me, sharing your own story of loss just when I needed it most.

Patricia Perez spent hours of tireless transcribing, and Donna Rice converted countless files into pdf format. They both kept Rep One sailing smoothly while I focused on writing. Thank you Patricia and Donna for being the kind of friends we all need more of.

Jill Fonseca read the first chapters of the manuscript in raw form and had the courage to ask for more. Thanks Jill for all the kitchen table encouragement while my kids raided your cookie jar. I couldn't ask for a better neighbor.

Many friends read the first draft of this manuscript and provided enthusiastic feedback: Karen Ferguson, Angela Loveless, Yolanda Lozano, Lynne Schwartz, Ivonne Theiss, Kimberly Thompson, Kathy Wilson, and Kathy Wishnew. Thank you all for your time and support.

My dear friend Jessica Prince asked me in Kindergarten, "Do you want to be my friend?" I'm glad I said yes. I want to thank you and everyone else who ever asked, "How's the book coming along?" You all know who you are.

Thank you to Cathi Lammert, RN, Executive Director of Share Pregnancy and Infant Loss Support from 1992-2007, for your selfless dedication to Share and the bereaved families who have found their way out of the storm because of your guiding light. Your support, encouragement and friendship mean more to me than I can express with words.

Many passionate women dedicated to the healing of bereaved families took time out of their busy schedules to read the manuscript including Lorraine Ash, author of *Life Touches Life: A Mother's Story of Stillbirth and Healing*; Joanne Cacciatore, Executive Director of M.I.S.S. Foundation; Jean Kollantai, Executive Director of CLIMB (Center for Loss in Multiple Birth); Perry-Lynn Moffitt, co-author of *A Silent Sorrow: Pregnancy Loss—Guidance and Support for You and Your Family*. Thank you all for your honest, invaluable feedback and encouragement.

Thank you agent Natasha Kern for caring enough about this project to send me in the right direction.

I am grateful to the universe for bringing Sharon Wesch and Jane Francis into my life just at the right moment. I often tell people my book shows the human side of pregnancy and infant loss. Sharon's and Jane's book-in-progress reveals the spiritual side of this important, yet misunderstood topic. Thank you, dear friends, for your inspiring work, your collaboration, and for connecting me with the people at Inkwell.

Nick Ligidakis at Inkwell Productions agreed to publish this book without reading a single word of the manuscript, relying solely on his instinct to sense my passion and energy for this story. I am amazed and humbled by his trust and belief in me.

Magon Kinzie, editor extraordinaire, put the finishing touches on this labor of love that was nine years in the making. I asked the universe to send me the perfect editor, and it delivered Magon. Thank you for your enthusiasm, skill, and wisdom (and your patience with all the *thats*). I am blessed to have had the opportunity to work with you.

John Meneely at Biltmore Pro Print did a fantastic job typesetting and never once complained about the countless changes I e-mailed him. Kelly Axtolis captured phenomenal photographs of flying fluffs (a.k.a. cottonwood seedlings) while on her stomach in a bed of weeds. And Adam Mehlhaff took the time to listen to my ideas and came up with a fabulous book cover. Thank you all!

My dear Yolanda, your guidance, wisdom, friendship, and love have allowed me to walk this path with grace. Thank you for being you.

To Kathy Wilson, my original soul sister. Since the sixth grade, you've stood beside me every step of the way, never flinching during my darkest moments. One of these days soon, I'll show my gratitude with a trip to some place far away, just you and me—for a whole week!

I've been blessed with the two best parents a person could ever wish for. Thank you Mom and Dad for sitting alongside our grief despite your own, and for always believing in me.

Thank you to my brothers, Brian and Eric, for always remembering Miranda. I love you both so much, and I know you love me back.

My three living daughters, Alex, Casey, and Anna, have always kept their baby sister Miranda in their hearts, sharing their own story of her with friends, teachers, Girl Scout leaders, and anyone else willing to listen. Thank you girls for your inspiration.

Finally, I want to thank my husband Al for walking this difficult path of grief with me. We didn't have a choice, but you never pulled away from me when I needed you most. And thank you for giving me the space to follow my dream. I love you.

Preface

"The quality of a person's life
cannot be judged by our limited understanding of time."

—from *When Hello Means Goodbye*
by Pat Schwiebert, RN and Paul Kirk, MD

I've become aware that you can ask anyone you know, and they have either lost a baby themselves or are close to someone who has. Pregnancy and infant loss has no boundaries. It does not discriminate based on religion, race, income, or any other factor. It affects all people, in all walks of life, all over the world, every day.

I found no comfort in being a statistic. Where I drew comfort, however, was from knowing that someone else on this planet understood my intense pain, the indescribable feelings of helplessness and loss. I drew comfort from knowing that other people had survived following the death of their own child, eventually finding happiness and purpose in their lives again.

Babies aren't supposed to die. Yet, each year, in the United States alone, approximately 26,000 babies are stillborn. Another 26,000 die within their first year of life. And it is estimated that nearly one million babies will be lost to miscarriage. Worldwide, these numbers become staggering. While pregnancy and infant loss affects millions of people each year, why are there still so many who know so little about it? Why are there so many people who are afraid to talk about it? Why are grieving parents expected to quickly "get over it" and get on with their lives?

My purpose is to give comfort, hope, and inspiration to those who have lost a child, and to foster understanding and compassion in those who are brought into the lives of the grieving or simply want to experience a powerful story of relearning to love life after loss.

Just as with the issues of infertility and postpartum depression, the time has also come to shatter the myths and taboos of pregnancy and infant loss. I wrote *The Good Grief Club* with the intention of shedding light on this subject, for where there is light there is healing and love.

Author's Note

The foundation of any support group is confidentiality, for it provides the basis for a safe environment in which to share our deepest thoughts, feelings, and experiences with honesty.

Every person's story in this book not only became a part of my own experience, but was shared enthusiastically with me in greater detail so that I could share it with you. The dialogue has been recaptured by those involved to the best of our memories. Many names are left unchanged with permission. However, some names have been changed to protect privacy.

~ ~ ~

A portion of the proceeds from the sale of this book will be donated to pregnancy and infant loss support programs.

"Without this great pain I would not have found myself capable
of truly loving what is lost
and by extension, what is still here."

—Lorraine Ash
from *Life Touches Life: A Mother's Story of Stillbirth and Healing*

1

I didn't see it coming. None of us did. How could we? For Heidi, Tracy, Wendy, and me, it came with the words, "There's no heartbeat." For Dawn, Beth, and Darlene, the crushing blow was, "There's nothing more we can do."

Between the seven of us, we have buried, cremated, or miscarried eighteen babies. Miscarriage, stillbirth, infant death—these were things that happened to other people. Until they happened to us.

This is our story.

~ ~ ~

It's the second Thursday of July, 1995. My husband, Al, and I make our way through an endless maze of hallways and elevators in the quiet north pavilion of Advocate Good Samaritan, the suburban Chicago hospital where both of our daughters were delivered. Now in the basement level, we pause outside the only open door in the long, deserted corridor. Looking at each other for strength, we take a deep breath and walk in. Our first support group meeting.

We're the first couple to arrive. Empty chairs are set up in a large circle; bright fluorescent lights glare down from overhead. Across the room in the corner is a woman setting out books on a table. Another woman, pretty and petite with shoulder-length dark hair, I guess to be in her 40s, is waiting to greet us. *That must be Pat Vaci, the Perinatal Support Coordinator,* I think to myself. Although she's never met us, she already knows who we are and introduces herself with a warm smile, embracing each of us. "Monica, Al, I'm glad you're both here. I'm sorry I wasn't there when you delivered Miranda. Candy stepped in for me while I was on vacation."

"We understand," I tell her. "Dr. Ross was disappointed you weren't there, but Candy was wonderful. She knew all the right things to say and do."

"Did you know Candy is new at grief work? She's never handled a full-term loss until yours."

"No, she didn't tell us, and I never would have guessed that," I answer. "I don't know what we would have done without her."

Pat smiles and nods. "Candy is a natural at grief work."

"I have the rest of Miranda's pictures for you," she says as she walks over to a table and comes back with a large envelope. I thank her and we sit down. I stare at the envelope, mustering courage to open it. Finally, I give in and open the flap, sliding out the pictures of my baby. Taking one look, I shove them back inside and quickly wipe the tears from my face.

We watch the door as people stream in. Some are couples like us, looking unsure, like students on the first day of school walking into the wrong class. Some women come in alone, others with a friend. I walk over to get a cup of juice and straighten my baby angel pin—anything to pass the time while nervously waiting for the meeting to begin. The air-conditioned room is, like most public buildings in the summer, too cold for me, and I'm glad I've worn Capri pants, albeit maternity. But I didn't think to bring a sweater to wear over my short-sleeved oversized shirt, and goose bumps are making their way up my arms. When I sit back down, Pat takes a seat next to me.

"Did all of these people deliver here at Good Sam?" I whisper to Pat.

"Some of them did," she answers. "But many of them delivered at other hospitals and were referred to us by someone."

Suddenly I remember something Candy told me during my hospital stay.

"Pat, you lost a baby too, didn't you?"

"I did," she answers quietly. "Our first child, Jennifer, was still-born at 38 weeks."

"I'm sorry."

"It was seventeen years ago. My husband and I were very private people and kept our grief to ourselves. There wasn't any support available that we knew about. We have two boys now." Sensing that she doesn't want the conversation to focus on her, I silently nod and cease my inquiry.

The circle is almost full with about a dozen or more people, and Pat announces that we'll begin. She reads the group's ground rules: "Everyone's grief is unique. There is no timetable for healing after a loss. No one will be asked to speak, but all are encouraged to share their feelings and experiences. Tears are outward signs of the depth of love. Here they are accepted, encouraged, and supported. If a group member needs to leave, someone will go along to be sure the person is doing okay and able to drive home. Confidentiality is an important aspect of group. Members are asked not to use the names of people or institutions in discussions inside or outside of group."

Pat asks a woman named Dawn to begin. She's tall, with dark medium-length hair and glasses and seems to be in her mid thirties. She's a veteran at this, I can tell. A few minutes ago, I watched her quietly laughing with some friends. "I'm Dawn. In February of 1994, I delivered triplets at twenty-three weeks. Christopher was pronounced dead after one minute. Katlyn lived for two days and Amanda lived for three days."

As I listen to Dawn talk, I'm amazed that after all she's been through she can sit here calmly and tell her story without tears. Although I can't see her battle scars, for they're hidden deep in her heart, I can tell with one look that her wounds have mostly healed. She's a survivor, and I find simple reassurance and hope from her.

After listening to several heartbreaking stories and watching tissue boxes being passed down the line, Al turns to me, his face overcome with emotion. I haven't seen him like this since the memorial service. "I can't believe we're here," he whispers. I nod. I know. Being in this room with these people validates our loss.

"I'm Beth," says a woman with short, brown hair wearing baggy shorts and a plain cotton shirt—like me, having just given birth and still stuck between maternity clothes and her prepregnancy wardrobe that doesn't fit yet—who looks about my age, mid to late twenties. "Last month I went into premature labor with my son Joshua. I was admitted to the hospital and given medication to stop the contractions, but I developed an infection, and the contractions kicked in again, and on June 19th Joshua was born at twenty-four weeks. Two hours later, he died in my hands. This is my first meeting," she says bitterly.

The woman sitting next to Beth, who came in with her, is now staring down at an imaginary spot on the floor in the middle of the circle. Also about my age, dressed in baggy post-maternity like Beth, with short, strawberry blond hair, her face becomes flush as she struggles to keep her composure. "I'm Heidi." Several seconds go by. I hold my breath. Finally she gathers the courage to speak, breaking the awkward silence. "I was thirty-two weeks pregnant with my daughter, Brittany. My five-year-old son, David, and I were on vacation in Florida with my mom and grandma. When I noticed the baby wasn't moving, I went to a nearby hospital. They told me there was no heartbeat. I flew home and two days later, on June 7th, my doctor induced labor and I delivered Brittany stillborn." Heidi wipes the tears from her eyes with a tissue and blows her nose.

Pat nods to me, signaling our turn. The women have been doing most of the talking, and when I turn to Al, he gives me a look of encouragement, holding my hand tight. "My name is Monica, this is my husband, Al. On June 20th, our daughter Miranda was stillborn at full term." I begin to cry and Al squeezes my hand harder. I hadn't expected it to be this difficult. The room is silent, heads nodding in understanding, as I struggle to catch my breath. "She had a knot in her cord." I hang my head down and grab a tissue out of the box that someone has handed me.

After introductions, the session becomes an open forum, and everyone is invited to talk about anything they're feeling. I don't know if I can talk. Maybe tonight I'll just listen.

"After my first miscarriage," says one mother, "I didn't even know if I should tell anyone other than a few close friends and relatives. The general attitude seemed to be that it's nature's way of taking care of something that wasn't supposed to be. Even though I didn't believe that, I tried to tell myself that maybe I shouldn't be so sad. But then when I had a second miscarriage, the pain of the first loss was compounded. I never really dealt with the grief, and now that I've lost two babies, I just can't pull myself together. Those were my babies. It doesn't matter how small they were. They were supposed to grow big and be born and we were going to be a family." The woman hangs her head down and cries quietly while the woman next to her reaches over and squeezes her hand.

I feel a sudden pang of guilt. I'm one of those people that had taken the "nature's way" attitude. Never having had a miscarriage, I hadn't considered the feelings of loss and helplessness a woman might feel if she deeply wanted to be a mother. I never thought about her hopes and dreams, and of the attachment she might feel to her newly forming baby. I should have known. I was attached from the moment I conceived both of my children. In fact, I was attached to the very idea of my daughters long before their tiny hearts ever beat for the first time.

The woman sighs and looks up again. "I still remember the day six months after my first miscarriage. I turned the calendar that month, and there it was, written in big red letters—BABY'S DUE DATE!

I fell apart all over again, like the miscarriage had just happened. When my husband came home and saw my red, puffy face, I pointed to the calendar. He didn't know what to say, so he just held me while I cried."

"I can't stop asking, Why? Why did this happen to me?" cries Heidi.

The room remains silent. We've all asked the same question countless times, and nobody has a good answer. Pat sits listening quietly, speaking only when asked.

"People I respected at my church told me it was God's will," says Beth. "It's part of God's plan, you'll learn something from this, God doesn't give you more than you can bear! So what is God's role in our everyday life? What makes someone else's prayer heard and not mine? We desperately prayed in the hospital, *Please, God, don't let our baby die!* But Josh died. Were my prayers unheard because they weren't said correctly? I feel like God didn't listen to my pleas, and I blame Him for taking Josh away."

"I asked the same questions you are," says Dawn. "People around me were praying to God, having faith that God would help them and take care of their problems. I was made to feel that if I went to church and prayed, bad things wouldn't happen to me. But where was God when I needed Him? We prayed harder in those few days at the hospital than at any other time in our lives. So many people were telling us, 'This was God's will.' It was one of the things I hated to hear the most. Why would God take away three babies from loving parents who wanted these children more than anything, yet allow a cocaine addict to have her baby only to let it suffer?"

I sit quietly, remembering Pastor Needham's words at Miranda's memorial service. He said that if he believed God had caused Miranda to die, taking away the life that I carried for nine months and which I grew to love even before she was born, he could not stand in his pulpit and speak to us. "I don't think God took my baby," I tell the group. "I just can't figure out why He didn't do anything to stop it."

"Our priest told us He's there, even though He may not be answering our prayers the way we want Him to," says Dawn. "And I said, 'Well, what good is He doing me then?' He told me God didn't want my babies to die; don't let people make me think that God took my babies away from me. Well, when I get up there and finally meet God, whoever is behind me in line is going to have to sit and wait for a long time, because He has a lot of explaining to do!" Everyone laughs, and for a moment the sadness is lifted. I wonder if Dawn realizes how funny she is without even trying.

The meeting goes on with issues that seem to be common to most of us. Birth story details. Funeral comparisons. Frustrations with unsympathetic medical personnel, family, or friends. More unhelpful things that well-meaning people say.

"Someone told me, 'You're young. You'll have more children,'" says Dawn. "Why do people say this? If they lost a parent, would it be okay for me to say, 'You're young, you can go find another parent'? Family members were telling us 'enough is enough, get on with your life, what's your problem, what are you moping around for?' People seem to think I didn't have time to get attached to my babies, that it shouldn't take me long to get over losing them. Because I never brought them home, some people act like it was no big deal. Would it bother them more to lose an older child than a younger child because the younger one wasn't around as long?"

"And then there are the ones who don't even remember and ask how the kids are doing," Dawn continues. "What I'd like to say is, 'Oh, well, they're six feet under. They're pretty dead by now.' I bite my lip trying not to laugh out loud, and glance around to see everyone else hiding grins and chuckles while Dawn goes on. "But instead, I just smile politely and tell them, 'Our children passed away. I don't know if you remember.' And then their eyes pop open, they apologize and walk away very quickly."

Dawn's had more than a year to deal with these issues and it's obvious. I wish I wasn't here, and I wish Dawn wasn't here, but at the moment I'm thankful for this woman with wisdom who shares my fate.

Heidi complains about the phone calls that come in. "'Congratulations, this is Olan Mills, your baby is one month old today. Blah, blah, blah.' At first I was nice about it and told them, 'Oh, I'm sorry, my baby died.' But after a while, I started yelling, 'You idiot! How dare you assume that my baby is healthy enough for a picture!'" Everyone laughs again, and I'm starting to get a sense that I've come to a very healing place.

Someone else complains about the endless stream of ads and coupons for baby products that began showing up in her mailbox after her baby's due date had passed. One woman received formula samples.

"There's a way to get your name off those lists," says Pat. "I'll give you the information after the meeting."

Beth tells us about a recent incident a few weeks ago. She was in a grieving haze; she didn't know the day or the time. She didn't know if she had even eaten that day. At a grocery store, on the way to her family reunion, she got into the express lane with one item and took out her debit card.

"Oh, well I guess this isn't the Cash Only line!" the woman behind her quipped.

Beth looked at her card as the cashier handed it back to her. She looked up at the sign. CASH ONLY. She looked back down at the card and then back at the cashier. "I thought this card was like cash," she said to the cashier.

"No, it's not!" snapped the woman behind her.

"No, it's not," sneered the cashier.

Beth began to cry. "You know what? I just buried my son! I'm sorry if I didn't read your damn sign!" she yelled. "You people are so damned inconsiderate." Now she was sobbing.

"I'm sorry," mumbled the woman behind her.

Beth grabbed her bag in an angry rage, went out to her car, and sat crying hysterically. She was so mad she could have punched someone. There was nothing she could do about the woman behind her. But she could do something about that cashier.

She marched back in and asked for a manager. "I spend a lot of damn money in this store, and I really don't deserve to be treated like this a week after I buried my son. I can't control what that woman behind me said, but I certainly have something to say about what your employee said to me. We can't all be perfect all of the time, and your employees need to know how to treat customers!" she sobbed.

"I'm so sorry!" the manager apologized. "Don't worry, I'll take care of this. We've had this problem before."

"Good, I hope you will!" she said and stormed out, glaring at the cashier who was watching. Beth felt good. She felt empowered. She was glad she hadn't punched anyone.

The room breaks into laughter and applause from those of us who envy Beth's courage, and as I watch the corners of her mouth curl into a grin, I get the feeling that, like Dawn, her brutal honesty is probably more humorous than she intended or realized.

At the end of the meeting, everyone is invited to stay and browse through the lending library books or talk with each other. I walk over to the table and scan the books covering a range of topics on death, grieving, pregnancy and infant loss. I grab two books—one on stillbirth, the other a collection of letters from bereaved parents—and wander over to Beth and Heidi. It's become apparent to me during the meeting that Beth and Heidi were friends before their losses, and I ask them to explain.

The two women knew each other casually through their husbands who went to high school together. When Beth learned that Heidi's baby, Brittany, had died, she was afraid of upsetting Heidi at the funeral with her own bulging pregnant belly, so she stayed away and instead sent Heidi a card.

Twelve days later, Beth's baby, Joshua, died. This time, Heidi sent Beth a card and wrote, *If you ever want to talk, just call.* Beth never called. One week later, Heidi called Beth. *Heidi will be so much better than me, I'm sure she'll have good things to tell me,* Beth thought, knowing Heidi was three weeks past Brittany's death. As Beth sat listening to Heidi go on and on, deeply immersed in grief, she thought, *She's not really doing so well. Is this what I sound like? Is this what I have to look forward to? I'm in big trouble.*

Heidi called again with information about a support group called Share, for pregnancy and infant loss, and asked if Beth wanted to go. "Greg isn't interested in going with me because he's healed," Heidi said. Beth laughed. Her husband, Jeff, wasn't like that; he wanted to talk about Joshua. He would have talked more about his son, but Beth was so incapable of supporting him that she didn't want to hear him talk about it. She didn't have it in her to take care of herself, let alone Jeff.

I nod my head, fully understanding. That's how I feel about my mom and mother-in-law; I can't bear their pain simultaneously with my own.

After talking with Heidi and Beth for a few moments, I already feel a bond with these two mothers. We all seem surprised at the intensity of the love and grief we carry for babies we knew such a short time. Having lost our babies within two weeks of each other, our grief is at the same stage and will likely coincide in the months to come. I realize I've found a new family in this circle of chairs; I'm not alone anymore. With every telling of my story and every tear shed, a tiny piece of my broken heart is mending.

We hug each other tightly and say goodbye until next month. Al and I slowly navigate the hallways and elevators, finally emerging outside into the parking lot, now dark. As we pull away, I look up at the five-story hospital. A wave of emotion overtakes me, and I'm flooded with the memory of the night one month earlier when I arrived here, scared and alone.

2
———

It was the third week of June, 9:00 on a Monday night—the night before my due date. I had settled into our living room rocking chair to eat a bowl of ice cream, having just put our two-year-old daughter, Alex, to bed. This was my nightly routine. I waited for the familiar kicks and jabs that came on strong this time every evening.

But that night they didn't come.

I finished my ice cream and stretched out on the couch like a beached whale. My belly responded with stillness. I pushed up and heaved my body over to the other side, waiting quietly. Still nothing. I knew babies often settled in as they neared birth. *The baby is probably just sleeping,* I tried to reassure myself. Nervously, I poked and prodded at my tummy, yet could feel no sign of movement. "Wake up, baby. Please wake up for momma," I whispered. The baby didn't answer. A deep ache filled the pit of my stomach and numbness began to course through my body as I replayed the day's events, frantically trying to recall the last time I had felt the baby move.

Al, who had been working upstairs in the loft, came down and sat on the couch, taking only a moment to notice the look on my face. "What's wrong?"

"I can't get the baby to move."

"You should call Dr. Ross."

That thought had already crossed my mind a dozen times, but it was late and I didn't want to bother him at home. Besides, he was on vacation, not on call. I wasn't even sure he was in town, but I had been with Dr. Ross long enough to know he would be upset if I was having a problem and didn't call him. I finally gave in to reason and nervously dialed the phone, hoping he was still home and still awake. The phone rang and rang and rang.

"Hello," his wife answered. I took a deep breath and asked if her husband was home.

"Hello." He sounded groggy.

"Dr. Ross, it's Monica Novak. I'm sorry to call so late, but I haven't felt the baby move in over an hour. The baby is always active at night. I'm getting a little nervous."

"There's probably nothing to worry about, but just to make sure, you really should go over to the Birth Center and have them check you out."

I promised to go and hung up with a temporary feeling of relief.

"He wants me to go to the hospital Birth Center," I told Al.

"Do you want me to take you?"

"No. I don't want to wake Alex up. I'm sure everything is fine. I'll be back in half an hour." He was worried and I was worried and I was trying to convince us both that nothing was wrong. I pulled out of the driveway wondering if I had made the right decision to go alone and then reminded myself that bad things didn't happen to me.

The ten-minute drive to the hospital seemed to stretch into an endless race. My dash lights were off, adding to my growing panic, but I was too nervous to find the switch and turn them back on. "Damn it!" I yelled, pounding on the dashboard. I opened the window letting the warm summer breeze blow in and fumbled for the radio, trying to calm myself with music.

When I walked through the double doors of the Birth Center, I was surprised to find the nurses expecting me, apparently having been notified by Dr. Ross. I followed a nurse into a birthing room and slid up onto the delivery bed.

"Are you having any unusual or bloody discharge?"

"No."

"Have you leaked any amniotic fluid?"

"No, I've just had light cramping on and off for a few days."

She put an external fetal monitor belt across my belly and began searching for the baby's heartbeat. I watched the clock. One minute passed. Nothing. She adjusted the belt. Another minute went by. The monitor picked up only the sound of the blood rushing through my veins. She readjusted the belt. The ticking of the clock echoed in my head. Still no heartbeat.

"Should I start worrying?" I asked as calmly as I could manage.

"No, not yet. The baby is probably just in a funny position. Sometimes it takes a while to find it." She hooked me up to a fetal doppler monitor, scanning my belly with a handheld wand, and made small talk while five more minutes passed. *It's never taken this long.*

Another nurse walked into the room to check our progress. My nurse looked at her and shook her head. "We're going to move you into a different room so we can do an ultrasound." I forced the fear from my mind, forced myself off the bed and followed her across the hall into another birthing room.

As she helped me up onto the bed, Dr. Ross suddenly walked in. "Get the ultrasound over here," he ordered. I was relieved to see him but realized I could no longer deny the possibility that something was terribly wrong. He turned on the machine and scanned my belly in search of the heartbeat. I began shaking. "Where's Al?" he asked.

"At home. With Alex." *Oh God, why did I come alone?* Holding my breath, my eyes jumped nervously from the monitor to his face for some sign of what was happening, the nurses standing silently behind me. It took only a moment for him to locate what he was looking for. His hand came to a halt and I waited for the unbearable silence to break.

"There's no heartbeat," he said, his eyes steady on the monitor.

My heart jumped. "You found the heartbeat?" I cried out with relief, my mind refusing to believe what my soul already seemed to know was true.

"No," he said quietly, looking down at me. "There is no heartbeat."

No heartbeat. His words buried me like a load of cement, and suddenly I was fighting to breathe. Head spinning, heart pounding, my body shook uncontrollably as shock set in. *No. This can't be happening. My baby…*

"I'm so sorry, Monica." He put his arms around me and I buried my face in his chest as violent sobs exploded from deep within.

"No! Why, why?" He had no answer and held me tight.

Minutes later I caught my breath, becoming quiet and still, looking down at the lifeless lump of flesh I had watched grow for nine months. He picked up the telephone next to the bed and asked for my phone number. A moment later, I listened to Dr. Ross tell Al the baby had no heartbeat and that he needed to come to the hospital right away.

~ ~ ~

I sat in my room waiting for Al, staring at the wall, hands on my stomach, stroking back and forth, hoping for some sign of life, desperately praying they had made a mistake and my baby was still alive.

The pregnancy had been fine, other than morning sickness which defied its name and lasted morning, noon, and night during the entire first trimester. Busy keeping up with a toddler, the months flew by, and by January, I was sharing the steady thumps of my kicking baby with Daddy and big sister. Although my world didn't revolve around this pregnancy as it had with my first, I often contemplated the changes a new baby would bring into our lives.

By the third trimester, the extra weight was taking its toll on my back, and I was grateful for my desk job as a data analyst for a health care system, where I spent twenty hours each week sitting at my computer, secretly counting down the days until I had the baby and would quit working to stay home with my two children. In the meantime, I treated my back to frequent baths, my belly sticking out of the water like a barren island, watching the waves ripple from the forceful kicks and rolls of the soon-to-be-born baby I was certain was a boy.

No heartbeat. But I heard it, just days ago, at my last prenatal visit—a strong heartbeat.

No kicking. Yet I felt it, just yesterday, driving home from Indiana—Father's Day spent with grandparents, aunts, uncles, cousins, brothers, everyone buzzing with excitement about my impending delivery—the baby deciding it was the perfect time to practice kickboxing while I held onto my belly and flashed a smile at Al. We were finally close to having this baby, the perfect gift for Father's Day—

Al rushed into the birthing room, jarring me from my memories, came to my side, dropped to his knees, and buried his head in my chest as we broke down sobbing in each other's arms. "Oh, God," he said.

"I don't know what happened," I cried

"What are we going to do?"

"I don't know," I answered, clinging to my husband for life.

A new nurse came into the room, bringing us water and offering her condolences. After we had spent time alone, Dr. Ross came in and sat down with a sigh.

"You need to make a decision. I need to know how you want to deliver this baby."

Al and I looked at each other and then back at Dr. Ross with blank, tear-stained faces. *We weren't prepared for this. How can we make decisions now?*

As I approached the ninth month, Dr. Ross and I had discussed my delivery in detail. He was going on a long-overdue extended vacation, and I was going to start seeing the other doctors in his group. "If I'm in town when you go into labor, call me and I'll come in to deliver you," he had said, handing me a slip of paper with his home phone number, pager number, and travel dates. Because I wasn't able to push Alex out, we were concerned that this baby might become too big, and we wanted to avoid another c-section. We agreed that if I hadn't gone into labor by June 23rd, three days after my due date, he would come in and induce labor, knowing he'd be back in town by then. I never made it to June 23rd.

Now everything had changed, and realizing we were going to need help with this decision, Dr. Ross continued. "You have three options. You can go home and wait for labor to start on its own—"

"No, I can't do that." I couldn't bear to carry my dead baby indefinitely, watching the minutes tick by until my body decided it was time, facing the constant, "When are you due?" from curious strangers.

"Okay, another option is that we can induce labor and see what happens," he said.

I immediately thought of Al's cousin Jeff and his wife Rachel in Iowa. After her first pregnancy had ended in miscarriage at eleven weeks and left her devastated, she and Jeff were expecting another new baby. It was two winters ago. The nursery was decorated, ready and waiting for afternoon naps and late night feedings. Something went wrong and the baby died. Rachel went through three days of hell, laboring to deliver her full-term stillborn son, whom they named Sean.

"Or we can do a c-section," said Dr. Ross.

I closed my eyes and thought of Rachel as I ran the options through my mind. Why should I labor for a baby who's not even breathing? I wanted this baby out now. I needed to know what happened. I had already had one c-section.

"What would you do if you were in this situation?" I asked, opening my eyes.

Dr. Ross looked at me intently. "If it were my wife, I would want to get through this as quickly as possible and find out what happened to the baby. After what you went through trying to deliver Alex, I would opt for the c-section. If you decide that's what you want, I'll stay here with you as long as it takes to get you into surgery." I didn't want another c-section, but now it seemed the only choice I was willing to make. Al agreed, and Dr. Ross left to make preparations for surgery.

A nurse came in and said Al's mother was out in the hall.

"What is she doing here? She's supposed to be home with Alex," I turned to Al, feeling a rush of mixed emotions. We had all the pain we could handle and couldn't bear hers too.

"It's okay. My dad is with Alex," Al told me and nodded to the nurse to let her in.

She hugged us each, crying, and sat on the edge of the bed. "What's happening? Is everything okay?"

"It's too late. We lost the baby," Al told her.

"No," she sobbed, "not to you, this can't happen to you! Why? What happened?"

We told her we wouldn't have any answers until we delivered the baby. After a short time we asked her to go and wait for our phone call.

It was midnight when Dr. Ross came back. The anesthesiologist on duty was tied up with an emergency appendectomy, and we wouldn't be able to get into surgery for two more hours; all we could do was wait, much like the night, two years earlier, when I had sat in a birthing room waiting for surgery to deliver Alex.

February winds whipped through us that day as we arrived at the hospital nervous and excited about bringing our first child into the world. I was surprised and relieved to see Dr. Ross already waiting for us in the Birth Center in the early morning. Hours later, when labor wasn't coming on its own, and my risk of infection was growing because of my leaking water bag, Dr. Ross induced the contractions. One of the nurses whispered that he was the only doctor who insisted on starting the medication himself and continued monitoring it throughout labor. I'd heard stories of nurses and residents managing labor only to have the doctor stroll in just as it was time to push the baby out. But Dr. Ross worked as hard as everyone on staff, staying with me until I held Alex in my arms late in the night after her delivery via c-section.

"Mr. and Mrs. Novak?" I was shaken from my memory by a new nurse who came in and introduced herself as Alice. Seeing our tears and distress, she brought more water and told us how sorry she was. I was prepped for surgery and signed the consent forms. Alice asked if we wanted a chaplain to be called in. We looked at each other and nodded. Dr. Ross checked in to make sure the nurses were taking good care of us.

Chaplain Lois arrived at 1:00 a.m., sitting down and saying a prayer for us and the baby. I didn't remember her words, only that she stayed, holding our hands, waiting.

~ ~ ~

At 1:30 a.m. I was wheeled to the operating room on a transport bed while Al was instructed to put on scrubs and meet us in the O.R. My body was shaking. I wanted this to be over with. At the same time, I knew delivering this baby would bring with it the reality of what I had lost. I wasn't ready to acknowledge that reality. How could I give up this child inside me along with the hopes and dreams I had for him or her?

The operating room was cold and bright. I was lifted onto the narrow operating table, and the anesthesiologist came in to administer the epidural which would numb the lower half of my body, allowing me to stay awake and alert during the delivery. I was rolled onto my side still shaking, knowing I had to keep completely still while the long epidural needle was inserted into my spine. I looked up at the nurse standing next to me. "Will you please hold my hand?" I asked her. She looked down, took my hand and gave it a squeeze. Biting my lip, I held my breath as I felt the pinch and slow sting. Several minutes later, I was rolled onto my back, legs strapped down, and waited, staring up at the ceiling as Al stroked my head. Without my contact lenses, everything around me was a blur.

Dr. Ross introduced me to his nurse, JoAnn, who was now standing at my side looking down at me. Although her face was hidden behind a surgical mask, I could see the compassion in her eyes.

"JoAnn came in to assist with your delivery," he told me.

"Thank you for getting out of bed," I said to her with a smile.

"You're welcome," she said and gently laid her hand on mine.

Suddenly I became lightheaded and the room began to spin. "Are you okay?" asked JoAnn.

"I'm dizzy, I think I'm going to pass out—"

"Get her some oxygen," said Dr. Ross. A few moments later, I stabilized and Dr. Ross asked if I was okay. I nodded.

"We're ready now, Monica. You shouldn't feel anything," he said. I felt a cold trickle of blood run down the side of my abdomen, but no pain. He worked to get the baby out, tugging and pulling. Al was sitting at my side holding my hand, and I stared up again at the ceiling with anticipation and dread. *Is it a boy or a girl?* I wondered. *Why did our baby die?* If there was no apparent sign of complication, we'd have to decide whether to do an autopsy. An image of my baby lying naked on a cold, metal examination table flashed before my eyes. I shuddered and forced it out of my mind.

The tugging stopped and I felt my body release its precious cargo. I waited for the familiar first cry of a newborn, but the room was silent and I was jerked back to reality.

"It's a girl."

Relief flooded over me. Suddenly I was laughing and couldn't stop. "I thought I was having a boy!"

"She's beautiful," said Dr. Ross.

"Look at the hair and those eyelashes," said JoAnn.

Now I was crying and couldn't stop. It was 2:06 a.m. on June 20th, 1995—my due date—and I had delivered a beautiful, dead baby girl.

Dr. Ross held up her umbilical cord and pointed to a tight knot halfway up. "The cord was wrapped around her neck and ankle, too. She looks really good and by her condition, I would guess that this occurred very recently, probably within the last 12-24 hours." With agreement from Dr. Ross, we decided against an autopsy. It was almost certain the knot in her umbilical cord had cut off her blood flow and, with it, her link to life.

Dr. Ross looked down at me. "Monica, this was a terrible accident." I wondered whether the cause of my baby's death made any difference. I hated the word "death." It wasn't right to use it in the same sentence as "baby."

I nodded and asked for statistics as if it might make me feel better to know how many other women shared this shocking fate. "One in one hundred babies are stillborn, half of those from cord accidents," Dr. Ross told me. The numbers were higher than I expected—26,000 a year in the U.S., I later learned. Stillbirth was more common than I realized. Still, how did I become that *one*?

"Where's Pat?" Dr. Ross asked one of the nurses as he stitched my abdomen together.

"She's on vacation this week."

I could see the disappointment in his eyes as he looked down at me. "Pat Vaci is a very special woman here who helps families with losses. I'm sure she'll be in touch with you, Monica, as soon as she gets back."

"Seven pounds, four ounces and twenty-one and a half inches long." Tears streamed down my face. *What does it matter now how much she weighs or measures?* A nurse asked Al if he wanted to hold the baby. Watching me struggle to stay calm, he shook his head no, too upset and focused on me, still flat on my back strapped to the operating table.

"We'll hold her in recovery together," he told her.

~ ~ ~

Thirty minutes later I was wheeled out to the recovery area where Chaplain Lois was waiting. It was the middle of the night, and the Birth Center was quiet. They propped pillows behind my back so

I could sit up. One of the nurses brought the baby out wrapped in a receiving blanket, laid her in my arms and pulled a privacy curtain around us. I dropped my lips to her head and brushed them against her soft, dark hair as tears fell onto to her still-warm skin. Crying, Al wrapped his arms around me and the baby. With my vision blurred and the pillows behind my back falling, I struggled to see her face clearly. But I knew she was perfect. We took turns holding her, passing her back and forth, reluctant to let go.

Before my pregnancy, as we contemplated another baby, I wondered how I could possibly love another child as much as Alex. Now I knew.

"Would you like to have her baptized?" Lois asked. We hadn't given this any thought, but at the moment it seemed the right thing to do.

"Have you decided on a name for her yet?"

We had chosen the name Samantha for a girl, Sam for short. I remembered the day we told my dad. "Alex and Sam? Great, then I'll have two granddaughters with boys' names," he had laughed.

I looked over at Al. "I want to save the name Samantha in case we ever have another girl."

"Then what are we going to name her?" he asked.

"Let's name her Miranda." It was my second choice. Miranda: Latin for admirable, beautiful, miraculous. Taken not from the daughter of Prospero in Shakespeare's *The Tempest*, but from the daughter of Shelly on CBS's *Northern Exposure*, my favorite show at the time.

Al gave his approval and Lois left to prepare for the baptism. In a few short hours, my baby had gone from a live Samantha to a dead Miranda.

Lois returned with a tiny white smock, stitched with a gold cross, and gently lifted it over Miranda's head. "Are you ready?" she asked. We nodded. "Lord our God, we are gathered together at this time to share our faith. We are overwhelmed as we reflect on the mystery of life and death, which we have just experienced. Father, you are the source of all life. We thank you for this little person—special, sacred and unique. Miranda Blair, I baptize you in the name of the Father, the Son, and the Holy Spirit."

"Into your hands, loving Father, we commend this child, Miranda Blair, to be with you in heaven forever. Al and Monica have loved this child. We pray your special blessing upon them. Give them strength and courage to accept this loss. Bless their family with a new bond of closeness as they grieve together."

An hour went by with more holding, hugging, kissing, crying. We had waited so long for this little baby and couldn't bear to say goodbye.

One of the nurses realized my struggle to let go. "She'll be kept here at the hospital until you decide what to do about a funeral, so you can hold her again later if you want." Al shook his head no, as if he had already made up his mind not to go through this again. I was leaning on him for strength, and if he couldn't handle it, how would I? Physically and emotionally exhausted, we told the nurse she could take Miranda.

"I love you," I whispered and gently kissed her forehead. As our baby girl was taken away, we watched in tears, believing we would never see or hold her again.

~ ~ ~

"What did you think of the meeting tonight?" Stopped at a red light, Al is looking over at me.

"What?"

"I said, what did you think of the meeting tonight?" he asks again patiently. He's gotten used to me disappearing into some distant place inside my head, having to repeat questions and wait longer than normal for a response.

"Oh, it was fine, I guess. It was hard. But I'm glad we went."

That night, after arriving home from the meeting emotionally exhausted, Al and I lie quietly, my head resting against his beating heart.

He touches me, stirring feelings deep inside that I haven't felt for a long time. My body responds, unable to ignore nature's primal instinct. Reality is suspended, Miranda blocked from our minds. We're in our own world, just the two of us, making love for the first time in months. It isn't passion as much as desperation; not a need for intimacy, but a cry for normalcy. For those few short moments in the dark, our lives feel normal again.

"I love you," I whisper.

"I love you too."

We collapse in each other's arms, sleeping well for the first time in weeks.

3

"Mommy?" Poke, poke. "Mommy, get up."

"It's too early, Alex. Go back to bed," I groan.

"Mommy."

"What."

"Get up."

"Alex, climb into bed with Mommy."

"No, Mommy get up!" Shake, shake.

If not for Alex needing me every morning, I would have no reason to get out of bed. I knew before I left the hospital that my life had changed in ways I couldn't yet comprehend. But it didn't fully hit me until the night I sat down with Al to watch *Seinfeld*, our favorite comedy. After five minutes I had to get up and leave the room. I couldn't even laugh at Kramer. I realized at that moment, my life as I knew it was over.

Since then, it's occurred to me that I'm indifferent to food—previously one of my main reasons for living—and activities I once considered fun hold no appeal. I can't watch any television, music makes me cry, reading requires more concentration than I can muster, and silence is unbearable. My life will never be the same, I'll never be happy again, and yet somehow the world and everyone in it continues on as usual. *Don't they know my child has died?* Of course not. But I want them to know. I want everyone to stop their lives and look at me. Stop having fun and cry with me. *Just stop!*

But my family and friends have gone back to their own lives, and I'm somehow supposed to go on with mine. Back to reality—grocery shopping, laundry, cooking, paying bills. *Who cares?* I struggle to get the simplest tasks done. Even playing with Alex is a chore. I stare at the walls, trying to make sense of everything. The walls stare back, saying nothing. The crisis is over, the food and flowers are gone, and I sit here with a two-year-old who hasn't a clue that life should be any different than it was before.

I suppose my grief is no different from anyone else's. It's just that very few people realize this, and even fewer know what to say. "Miranda's memorial service was really nice," said a friend on the phone one day. I remember her face, wet and red from crying, her compassion touching me as Al and I carried Alex towards the back of the church that morning. "I couldn't understand why I was so emotional, though," she continued. "Then I found out why. I'm pregnant! I always get really emotional when I'm pregnant." Stunned at her announcement, I managed to congratulate her, hurt that the tears I thought were for Miranda were, in truth, brought on by her new baby. Those words hurt, too. *Her new baby.*

Others attempt to comfort me with written words, and I've become accustomed to pulling a handful of shared sorrow out of the mailbox each day. Sympathy cards come from the most unexpected sources, like my ex-boyfriend and church members we've never met. But even the mail has its hazards, like the day I opened the first of many medical bills, an invitation to a friend's 4th of July party—as if I had something to celebrate—and a birth announcement from a friend whose wife and I recently commiserated together about our aching backs and the growing summer heat, agreeing that our deliveries couldn't come soon enough.

Through all of this, I know the focus has been, and still is, on me. Not only because I physically carried and lost the baby, but because I'm a woman. Al has lost a child too, but as a man, he's expected to be the strong one, to take care of me, Alex, and anything else that needs to be taken care of. I know he's hurting inside, but he doesn't express it openly, and I sometimes wonder if his lack of emotion means that he doesn't feel the loss I feel, that he doesn't care as much.

So I'm relieved when I answer a phone call from one of Al's old friends, hoping he'll finally get some of the support I've been getting from others. "I'm sorry about the baby," the friend says.

"Thank you," I say.

"You just have to get on with your life," he adds.

"Yeah, I guess you're right," I answer, rolling my eyes, and handing Al the phone. *You don't just get on with your life when your child has died. A guinea pig, yes, but not a child. Why is he giving me advice anyway? He doesn't have children. What the hell does he know?!*

There is one man I'm sure will know what to say to Al—his cousin Jeff. Although the causes of death differed—Sean's life, Jeff and Rachel learned several months later, was claimed by an antibody; Miranda's life ended with a cord accident—the grief is the same. It doesn't take much effort to convince Al to take a spur-of-the-moment trip to Iowa to see Jeff and Rachel.

On the six-hour drive to Des Moines, I pray this trip is better than the last trip we took. Just weeks after losing Miranda, my parents invited us on their annual summer trek to Hamlin Lake, in Ludington, Michigan. I hadn't been there since getting married and was grateful for the distraction and change of scenery. I welcomed the reprieve from loneliness and looked forward to fishing, swimming, boating, and spending time with my family.

Our escape to Michigan was not the perfect getaway I had expected. Despite the company of my family, I walked around with a cloud over my head, easily annoyed with little things everyone said or did. On the fourth day, I got into a shoving match with my youngest brother, and neither of us knew why. I wasn't myself—*who was I?*—and told Al I wanted to go home. As we pulled away, I watched my family wave, my mom on the verge of tears, until we were out of sight. Staring out the window, I shared her longing for the happy family times we once had, but as we headed back towards the loneliness and pain that awaited our return, I realized everything was different now.

Jeff and Rachel are waiting for us when we pull into their driveway late at night, and the four of us stay up for hours talking about Miranda and Sean. While I sit looking at Sean's photo album, Rachel asks if I have any pictures of Miranda. "I didn't bring them. It's too hard to look at them."

"You'll be ready for them some day," says Rachel.

I smile. "I hope so."

We share a few laughs, a few tears, and finally head up to bed.

"It's good to be here," I whisper to Al and drift off to sleep.

~ ~ ~

Al and Jeff leave early to play golf, and Rachel and I sit talking while Alex plays on the floor. I ask her to tell me more about losing Sean.

After the delivery, Rachel's blood pressure wouldn't stabilize and they kept her in the hospital for three days. The medical staff thought she was suicidal and assigned a nurse to keep guard over her every time Jeff had to leave.

Once home, she had to pass the baby's nursery full of new baby things. The room seemed foreign as if it didn't belong there. Her mom and sister wanted to put Sean's things away for her, but she told them she didn't want anyone in there. She shut the door and left it closed for three weeks.

Rachel's sister took over at home, having food catered from the grocery store. The baptism instructors from their church brought breakfast over and left it on the front porch one morning. They got flowers and cards from so many people. Rachel couldn't figure out how all of these people found out about Sean's death.

Rachel's brother was driving six hours each way to be with Rachel at the hospital in Des Moines, go back for his sons at home in St. Louis who were worried about Aunt Rachel, and then return to Des Moines with them for the upcoming memorial service. This was a brother who never called Rachel, but was there when she needed him.

Jeff's brother and his wife had, along with other family, driven six hours to Des Moines from Chicago. They had just given birth to a baby girl one month earlier, and although they had brought a video tape of the baby, they were reluctant to show it to Jeff and Rachel who hadn't seen their new niece yet, worrying that the video would be too upsetting. Jeff and Rachel insisted on watching it. The baby, with a full head of dark hair, was beautiful, and when Rachel began to cry, Jeff's brother jumped up to turn it off, but Rachel wouldn't let him. As hard as it was for her to watch, she and Jeff were thrilled for them and their new baby.

Rachel's sister ordered flowers for the memorial service and had Sean's hospital keepsake certificate framed, bringing it along with his hospital t-shirt to the church.

Jeff's brother videotaped the memorial service and set it to Eric Clapton's "Tears in Heaven," giving Jeff and Rachel a keepsake video of their own in memory of Sean.

Although she didn't know Jeff and Rachel, Sister Cathy from the church came to the service. She had also come to visit them in the hospital. And for months after, she called them to see how they were doing and tell them they were being prayed for. She never forgot.

Although Jeff and Rachel's family and community had rallied around them in their darkest hours, the pain and anger was swelling up around them. They drove to St. Louis for Thanksgiving, but didn't feel they had anything to be thankful for, and as Rachel's family members took turns around the table offering a prayer of thanksgiving, Rachel ran from the table crying.

Rachel's close childhood friend Tammy knew Sean had died and that Rachel was home at her mom's. Tammy came over with her girls, and Rachel sat listening about Tammy's week from hell, how she had been fighting with her mother-in-law, money was tight, her children had been sick, and her children were such brats, blah, blah, blah. Tammy stayed for an hour and then left, never mentioning or acknowledging Sean. Rachel was furious. *How could someone be so self-centered? All she needed to say was, "I'm really sorry about your baby, I wish I knew what to say, or I wish there was something I could do."*

Rachel's friend Laura, on the other hand, called every day. Laura sat and listened to Rachel talk for hours and hours, never once getting bored, irritated, distracted, or annoyed. Every time Laura saw Rachel, she hugged her and told Rachel she was still thinking of her and Sean.

Laura had given birth to a baby boy just five months earlier. Although Laura's baby was a sad reminder that Jeff and Rachel didn't have Sean with them, Rachel tried very hard not to take any joy away from Laura. Rachel loved going to Laura's house and being around her baby, and because Laura was such a wonderful friend, Rachel felt closer to her than she ever had before.

Jeff and Rachel were home again trying to pick up the pieces, with no direction, unsure of where they should be or what they should be doing. One night while Jeff was sleeping, Rachel went into Sean's room, sat in the rocking chair and rocked herself in the dark. *It's midnight, just about the time I would be feeding Sean.* She sat for an hour thinking and crying. It felt right to be there, yet so much was missing. She spent many nights in the nursery crying, rocking and looking out the window at the beautiful tree in the backyard thinking how unfair this was.

Jeff was back to work and Rachel was alone. She had no job, nothing to do, and depression set in. Her daily routine consisted of getting out of bed and lying on the couch watching television all day long, never leaving the house, her body putting on the pounds with each passing day. She was supposed to be taking care of her new baby; now she had no purpose, no reason to get up and do anything.

Frustration and anxiety built up inside Rachel until she could no longer hold it in and began throwing things across the room at a wall: books, a dish, anything she could get her hands on. When Jeff realized she needed an outlet, he bought her a treadmill, and she got on it every time the misery became too much. There were days when she was on and off the treadmill for hours, letting her emotions pour out of her. She acknowledged her depression and made a conscious decision to take control and wipe it totally out. *If I can look like I've never had a baby, I can feel like I've never had a baby, and then I won't feel so miserable,* she told herself.

She began dieting and quickly lost fifty pounds—she hadn't been so thin since high school—and her faith was strengthened. Whenever she began to feel overwhelmed and couldn't take it anymore, something would happen, like a phone call, to pull her out of it and boost her spirits. She knew there was a higher power looking over her, that she wasn't alone in this.

They still missed Sean deeply, but started talking about having another baby. It became a quest; they had to prove they could do it. "We're going to get pregnant, and we're going to have another baby, and we're going to do it now, and everything is going to work! Nobody is going to take this away from me and get away with it!" she announced to the universe.

Our conversation is interrupted by the sounds of a crying baby, and Rachel gets up and leaves the room. A moment later, she comes back holding eight-month-old Abigail, born thirteen months after Sean. "Can I hold her?" I ask. Rachel hands her beautiful baby girl to me. This is the first time I've held a baby since saying goodbye to Miranda. She's soft and her hair smells of baby shampoo. She sits in my lap playing with my fingers while I study her every feature. Alex makes faces at Abby, who quickly forgets about my fingers and squirms down onto the floor to investigate Alex's "big-girl" toys.

"Do you remember when we came to Chicago that New Year's Eve after we lost Sean and eight of us went out to a Mexican restaurant?" she asks me. I nod, remembering that we were all so afraid of upsetting them that nobody mentioned Sean. "Jeff got really drunk. We looked like we were handling everything fine on the outside. On the inside, we felt guilty for having what little fun we could muster. That same weekend, at a family birthday party, I spent the entire day crying uncontrollably upstairs. I couldn't bear to be around everyone, listening to them talk about their children and birthdays. There was nothing anyone could do for me. I cried the entire six hours back to Des Moines. When I got home, I realized I couldn't sit in this house any longer and wither away. So I decided to put my talent to good use and started sewing window treatments for people."

I smile and nod. "You know, people can't believe it when I tell them this happened twice in the same family," I tell Rachel.

"I couldn't believe it either," she says. "The day Jeff's brother called to say that you and Al had lost your baby, I kept asking, 'How's Monica? How's the baby?' He had to stop me and ask if I had heard what he had just told me. And then it hit me. He asked several more times if I understood what he was saying. It was like I couldn't accept it. *If I simply ignore it, it won't be happening,* I told myself. I thought we were over this. I felt so bad for you."

"What did you do with Sean's ashes," I ask Rachel.

"I couldn't bring myself to take his ashes home with me, so the funeral home kept them for a very long time. Three times during the next three months, I went to the funeral home and sat there with the small wooden box on my lap that contained Sean's remains. Finally, after many months, I brought the ashes home and put the wooden box on my fireplace mantel. Sometimes I lean over and kiss the top of the box, blow it a kiss, or lay my hand on it to feel close to Sean." I smile, looking up at the box on her mantel.

"Did you know Al's brother called Jeff and me to ask what you should do about Miranda's ashes?" she says.

"No, but I remember the conversation we had with him in the hospital."

"Have you decided what you're going to do with Miranda's ashes?" my brother-in-law had asked Al and me. I was touched by his concern for his niece's remains, but my numbness made it impossible to make rational decisions about what to circle on the lunch menu, let alone what to do with the ashes of my cremated baby.

"I guess we'll let the funeral home dispose of them," I answered blankly.

He told us that someday we might want Miranda's ashes, either to keep, bury, or scatter. He seemed to be making sense, and we nod-ded, but still had no answer for him. So he offered to take her ashes home with him until we could decide what to do. Grateful, we accepted. Now I realize it was thanks to Jeff and Rachel that he was able to counsel us through that important decision.

"How's Al doing?" she asks.

"I don't know. We don't talk about Miranda, and I never see him cry."

"I had the same experience with Jeff after Sean died. I could-n't understand why he never cried when crying was all I could seem to do. 'I do cry!' he yelled at me one day. 'I cry in the shower, and in my car on the way to work, and at night when you're asleep. I just don't want to talk about it all the time like you do!'"

Later, when the guys get home, Rachel asks Jeff if he and Al talked about Sean and Miranda. Jeff tells her no.

At the same time, Al and I are talking in our room, and I ask him the same question. He says no.

"Why didn't you ask Al if he wanted to talk about it?" she asks Jeff. Jeff shrugs.

"I thought you would take advantage of the time alone with Jeff to talk about the babies. That's all Rachel and I talked about," I tell Al. Al shrugs.

"Five hours together and no mention of either baby," I tell Rachel later, shaking my head.

"That just goes to show you how different men are, doesn't it?" she says.

At the end of the weekend, we hug each other tight and promise to stay in touch. On the drive home, I think about Rachel's answer when I asked how long it was after losing Sean that she started to feel better, to feel normal again. "I hit my lowest point about three months after Sean's death." Her words echo in my head. It hasn't even been six weeks for me. *How can things get any worse?*

4

It's the second Thursday of August. Al and I have come to our second support group meeting. We nervously walk in, but this time see familiar faces. Pat gives us each a hug. "I'm glad you're both here."

"This is for Share," I tell her, handing her an envelope containing a check for ninety dollars from people we've never met. "My dad's office took up a collection, and we want you to have it."

"Thank you," she says. "We can use it to buy new books for our library."

I remember to grab a handful of tissue on the way to an empty seat so I don't have to wait for the box to get around to me later. We sit down and I smile across the room at Beth and Heidi. I can tell they're as happy as I am to see Dawn walk in and sit down.

The introductions start, and we listen to stories from people who have lost their babies within the past month. Heidi, Beth, and I have already earned veteran status in comparison.

This time I get through the introductions without choking up and sobbing. Not so for a young woman named Darlene. She's young, with long brown hair pulled back into a tight pony tail, no make-up, and wearing sweat pants and a t-shirt. She gets her name out and then breaks down crying. A woman gets up and walks over to her. "I think you need a hug," she says and wraps her arms around Darlene.

A few minutes later, when Darlene has calmed down, she tells us she and her husband, Larry, lost premature twin boys the month before. "They didn't check for twins, so I wasn't treated as a high-risk pregnancy. I was doing regular things. I still think it was my fault because I went horseback riding. The doctor told me I could, he said I could do it all. Larry, my husband, said it's not my fault. But still, mothers need a reason, don't we? We have to blame somebody."

"I know what you mean," says Beth. "I blame myself for going into premature labor with Joshua. If I hadn't drunk a Coke, maybe I wouldn't have been dehydrated and gone into labor."

I look around the room and then back at Beth. "A Coke? Come on, Beth, do you actually believe that?" I ask. She smiles, and then laughs, and before long the entire room is laughing.

"I know, it sounds stupid, but that's what I've been telling myself," says Beth.

Someone asks Darlene if either of her twins survived the birth. "Nicholas was stillborn, but Nathan was alive. Only, they didn't tell us. We told them not to take any lifesaving measures because they told us there was no hope. So when he was born they took him away. He lived for two hours and we didn't even know it. He died alone. It was terrible. I don't know if they let him die because we told them not to do anything. Now I keep asking if Nathan would still be alive if we had told them to try. I never saw my doctor after they were born, and there was no communication from the hospital staff," Darlene cries.

"Then an old friend of mine, someone I've known since the second grade, called and when I told her I just lost my twins at five months, she said 'Really? Because I just had an abortion. I wasn't two months along like I thought, I was four months along. Tell me what your babies looked like so I'll know what mine looked like.' I had to get off the phone. I couldn't even talk to her."

"Doesn't that make you angry?" says Beth. "Some people are so clueless. Like this lady at the grocery store last week."

Oh no, not another one, I think to myself. *I hope she hasn't finally punched someone.*

Beth tells the group that one afternoon she and Madeline, her two-year-old, walked out of the grocery store, laughing and enjoying the moment together. When they stopped to unload the groceries in the trunk, she noticed another car parked only inches from her door.

The woman, still in her car, rolled down the window and began screaming at Beth. "It was really rude of you to park this way!"

"I'm sorry, I had to park that way because the car next to me was parked over his line," Beth apologized.

"Well, I'm pregnant and I can't get out of my car!"

She's been sitting there just waiting to yell at someone, thought Beth, feeling the anger well up. "You know what? My baby died and I hope yours does too!" Beth screamed, the words spewing out of her like hot lava. The woman quickly rolled up her window and backed out of the spot. "So maybe she didn't feel good. She should just be thankful she's pregnant."

We nod, some grinning, some giggling. "I remember what it felt like to be pregnant," continues Beth. "Pregnant people don't walk around thinking that their pregnancy could be hurting other people's feelings. They feel like the world should revolve around them. I know, because I felt that way during Madeline's pregnancy. They need to think about other people, too."

After a moment of silence, another mom speaks up. "I'm so sick of that stupid Hugh Grant movie *Nine Months,*" she complains. "I've been looking at billboards and commercials for two months and now everyone is talking about it." Everyone here agrees they would rather have their eyelashes plucked out one at a time than watch one hundred and three minutes of pregnant Julianne Moore's bulging belly.

Heidi tells us she just spent Brittany's due date at the cemetery. She and her mom sat under a golf umbrella in the 105 degree heat, next to a boom box, listening to a tape she made of songs, mostly lullabies, that reminded her of her baby. Crying, they wrote a letter to Brittany and sent it up to the heavens tied to a balloon.

Everyone smiles or nods at Heidi. The room becomes quiet, and everyone takes on their quiet habit. Either you stare at the floor—most of the men fall into this category—or you fidget with damp tissues shredded from constant wringing, or you glance from face to face, wondering who will speak next.

"I'm glad they didn't take away the pain of childbirth, because that was the last physical feeling Josh ever gave me," says Beth.

"I was glad I held Brittany, rocked her, sang to her," says Heidi. "But I wish I had undressed her. I wish I had bathed her. I didn't know to, no one directed me to."

"I have pictures of Miranda, but none of me or Al holding her," I tell everyone. "And I had my camera with me the entire time, but it never occurred to us to take a family picture, and nobody suggested it. Sometimes I wonder if I should have waited and delivered her later instead of taking her out by c-section in the middle of the night. Then our families could have been there. We could have taken pictures. We would have been more prepared."

"I found out, after looking at the medical records, that the hospital staff knew I was developing an infection long before they told me," says Beth. "If only I had known, I could have spent more time preparing for Josh's death; I could have found a book or pamphlet, gotten my camera, called family. Instead, I held onto false hope. When I brought this up with the doctors, their answer was, 'We can't do that because we don't know if the baby is going to live or die, and we don't want the mother to lose hope.' There should be a pamphlet for parents who are in limbo, something that says 'this is not to take away your hope, but here's what you can expect, this is what you can do, this is what is acceptable.'"

It dawns on me after listening to these women, and myself, that what happened or didn't happen during those crucial moments following the discovery, delivery, and death of their babies was a large factor in how they were handling their grief in the weeks, months, and even years that followed. Almost every one of us had regrets of not carrying out every possible act of mothering towards our babies that could have possibly been done. It was our one and only chance, and amidst the shock and confusion of what was happening, we relied heavily, almost solely, on caregivers and family members to guide us through this harrowing experience.

For those of us who had only hours with the babies we thought we would have a lifetime with, those minutes and hours suddenly replaced that lifetime and became the memories we would carry with us forever, and eventually, for many, would bring us peace or comfort in that remembering.

For those who had no time with their babies—the ones who miscarried or were discouraged from seeing their babies—well, where do they go with that pain if not to a place of memories? All that's left are the "what ifs" and "if onlys" of their dreams.

After the meeting, Al and I walk over to Pat. "Did Candy tell you about the two doctors who came into my hospital room and didn't know I had lost a baby?" I ask her.

"Yes, I heard about it," she says. "I'm so sorry that happened. The doctor who discharged you yelled at the nurses for not telling him you had lost your baby. After that incident, I started putting new cards on the doors of bereaved mothers that display the Share logo. It's a pair of hands cradling the heart, designed by a bereaved mother. We also put stickers with the same logo on the inside and outside of medical charts of women who have lost a baby. Then I posted the logo in key areas where housekeeping and volunteers will see it often. I spot-check staff to make sure they know what the logo means if they see it on the door of a patient's room." I nod with satisfaction, glad my experience will hopefully prevent additional distress for other mothers.

While Al browses at the books on the table, I spend a few minutes talking to Dawn who I've learned is a labor and delivery nurse here at the hospital. Then I wander over towards Beth and Heidi who are talking with the new woman, Darlene. "Larry had to work, and I was afraid of coming here by myself and looking stupid," she tells us. "I feel frumpy and didn't know how to dress. And I wasn't sure what people talked about at these meetings. When the introductions started, I was thinking I couldn't do it. But why was I here if I wasn't going to talk?"

"It was like that for us at our first meeting, too," says Beth.

"It gets easier," Heidi reassures her.

"And believe me, nobody here cares what you look like," I add. "This ain't no fashion show." Darlene smiles.

~ ~ ~

Why didn't I just wait until the next day? I ask myself on the drive home. *Why didn't I wait for my family? Why didn't we take photos with Miranda?* I didn't realize until tonight how differently I might have done things had I been prepared, or had Candy or Pat been there with us in the middle of the night. As the questions torment me, the memories come rushing back.

5

Tight pressure around my arm awakened me as I looked up at a nurse who was checking my vitals. I squinted at the clock—6:15 a.m., Tuesday morning. I had gotten ninety minutes of reprieve from my living nightmare. Had we really just delivered a baby girl? Had she really been stillborn? Was she really gone?

Al, who was asleep next to me on a cot, slowly sat up and looked around the room, my new home for the next three days. The recovery nurse had offered to put me on a different floor, away from other new mothers and their babies, but I told her no. I didn't want to deny that I had just given birth and knew I would get the best post-partum care here on the maternity floor. So she brought us to a private room at the end of a quiet hall, as far away from the nursery and crying newborns as possible.

Both awake now, it was pointless to try to go back to sleep, and I hadn't called my parents yet; knowing the mental state they would be in, I didn't want them making the one-hour drive from northwest Indiana to the suburbs of Chicago in the middle of the night. I was sick with anxiety at the thought of telling them their second grandchild had died without a chance to say hello. My heart was already pounding, and my hands shook as I dialed the phone.

"Hello."

"Dad, are you awake?" I asked, fighting to get the words out before I choked up.

"Yeah, I'm awake," he mumbled, half asleep.

"Is Mom with you?"

"Yeah, she's here."

"Dad, I'm in the hospital." I heard him whisper to my mom and suddenly couldn't hold back the tears anymore.

"What's wrong?"

"We lost the baby."

"What?"

"We lost the baby, Dad," I told him, now sobbing.

"Oh Moni, oh no! What happened?" My heart broke a little more at the sound of my dad crying. I had only seen him cry once before, when his father died.

"There was a knot in her cord."

"What?" said my mom.

"They lost the baby." My mom was crying on the phone now.

"How soon can you get here?"

She told me they would make some phone calls, pack their overnight bags, and be up as soon as they could. "I love you," she said.

"I love you too."

~ ~ ~

I've seen her somewhere before, I thought, as a woman walked into my room shortly after and introduced herself as Candy Sibly. She was attractive, about the same age as my mom, early to mid forties, I guessed. *I remember. She's a nurse and lactation consultant. I took her breast-feeding class when I was pregnant with Alex.* She told us she was filling in for Pat Vaci, Perinatal Support Coordinator, the one Dr. Ross told me about.

She sat and asked if we wanted to talk about what happened. I took a deep breath and began. "It was 9:00 Monday night and I was eating a bowl of ice cream…"

Candy listened patiently, holding our hands and encouraging us to cry when we needed to. She seemed perfectly comfortable with our pain, helping us talk through our experience and emotions.

"Do you want to see Miranda again?" she asked.

I sighed and looked at Al. "I don't know," I said, missing her already. "Will she be cold?" I asked. Candy was encouraging but explained, yes, our baby would be cold, part of her skin discolored. I was afraid to see and feel her that way and thought it might be best to rely on my memory of her in the recovery room. I was looking to Al for direction and strength, and he clearly didn't want to repeat the emotional upheaval of saying goodbye to our baby. "I don't think so," I told her.

"That's alright. Do whatever feels comfortable for you. There's no right or wrong here. But don't be surprised if you change your mind before you leave the hospital, and that's okay, too."

She told us about Share, a support group for pregnancy and infant loss that Pat facilitated once a month. "Do you think you might be interested in this?" I nodded my head and she handed me a pamphlet. We had just missed the June meeting and would have to wait another month for the next one.

"I have something else for you," she said, handing me a booklet. *When Hello Means Goodbye—A Guide for Parents Whose Child Dies Before Birth, At Birth or Shortly After Birth.* "It will help you plan the baby's funeral arrangements and guide you through the grieving process." *We weren't supposed to be planning a funeral, we were supposed to be putting a stork sign in the front yard! It's not fair that other families are going home with their babies and we're going to a funeral!*

"I'm so sorry. Are you okay?" she asked before getting up to leave. We nodded. "If you need anything at all, you can page me at any time of the day or night. If anyone else wants to hold the baby, just let me know. I'll be checking in later to see how you're doing." She squeezed my hand and gave a reassuring smile, leaving us alone with a booklet, a pamphlet, and an overwhelming amount of pain.

~ ~ ~

When my parents rushed into the room, I burst into tears. They sat on my bed, crying, holding their only daughter while I sobbed uncontrollably, unaware that I had been holding in emotions all morning until they could be here to comfort me, just like when I was a little girl. Except this time they couldn't make it all better.

After a few minutes, I caught my breath.

"Tell us what happened."

"It was 9:00 Monday night and I was eating a bowl of ice cream..." Once again I replayed the details of the night before. They held my hands, listening intently and asking questions.

"Do you want to see the baby?" I asked. They both answered yes. I called Candy and a few minutes later she walked in and introduced herself. "Can you please bring the baby up for my parents to hold?"

"Of course. Would you like me to bring her here to your room or take your parents to a private room to be with Miranda?"

I hesitated.

"A private room," Al told her, and my parents followed her out the door.

Everyone was calling Miranda by name—except me. I could only call her "the baby." That was how I had known her for the past nine months. She had only been Miranda for a few hours and her name sounded foreign to me. Hearing Candy and my parents call her Miranda gave her an identity. *What's wrong with me that I can't say my own baby's name?*

"What are we going to do about a funeral?" I asked Al. We had never planned a funeral—I could count my funeral experiences on one hand, mostly for distant relatives over the age of sixty—and Al and I hadn't even discussed our own plans with each other. I shuddered at the thought of my baby lying in a casket and began to cry again. "I can't bury her in the ground," I told him.

"What about Jeff and Rachel? What did they do for Sean?" Al asked.

"Sean was cremated and given a memorial service at their church." We agreed to do the same: cremation and then a memorial service at church on Saturday. On the phone, Pastor Needham, who had already been in that morning to see us, said Saturday would be fine and told us he would contact the funeral director.

~ ~ ~

My parents sat in a small office waiting for Candy to bring them their new grandchild. She soon returned, wheeling a bassinet into the room. Candy asked my mom if she wanted to pick the baby up herself. Fighting back the tears, she shook her head no and asked Candy to do it. Candy unwrapped Miranda from her receiving blanket, revealing a soft pink gown with white bunnies, and handed her to Mom. Rocking Miranda, mom cried and sang a lullaby. She couldn't bear that the baby was so cold and rubbed her hands up and down Miranda's tiny arms to warm her skin. She handed the baby to my dad and he cried.

When Candy came back to check on them, they asked for more time. Her little body was beginning to warm up, and Dad took her hat off to stroke her hair. "It's so strange," he said, "that she looks and feels like a live baby, but she isn't here."

"Look at her long pretty fingers," said Mom.

They noticed that Miranda had soiled herself with meconium—a baby's first bowel movement, not uncommon for a stillborn baby after delivery—and when Candy returned, she cleaned her up. She took a Polaroid of Dad holding Miranda, then two of Miranda with Mom. They laid the baby down in the bassinet and Candy took several more pictures.

An hour and a half later, my parents returned to my room, faces worn, eyes red and swollen.

~ ~ ~

Al's parents brought Alex that afternoon. She ran to my bed and climbed up. "Be careful, don't jump on Mommy!" everyone yelled.

I hugged her tight, but she wiggled loose, patted my stomach and said, "Baby in tummy." Towards the end of my pregnancy, I would pull Alex's hand to my belly so she could feel the baby move. As if playing a game of cat and mouse, her baby sister would stop kicking. The moment Alex got impatient and walked away, the kicking would start up again. *Alex come find me!* the baby teased. I'd call Alex back and the game would go on. That game is over.

Alex was only two and didn't understand what was happening. Hiding my emotion, I tried to explain that her baby sister wasn't in there anymore, but before I could get any further, she was off my lap and exploring the room. It was the first and last time she would ever say anything about the baby.

Al's parents asked to see Miranda and my dad took them down the hall to find Candy. When they returned twenty minutes later, Candy asked if we would like Alex to see her sister, but I told her I was afraid she might get scared or confused. I didn't know if I was doing the right thing, trying to protect Alex from a natural part of the life cycle, but it was the best I could do at the moment.

~ ~ ~

That night, I sat alone in my newly decorated room with pink floral curtains and wood floors, staring out the window into the darkness, wondering if I should have asked Al to spend the night with me. He offered, but I sent him home with Alex.

The day's events replayed in my head: family and friends calling to say they were sorry and ask how we were; nurses, medical techs, dietary clerks, and lab techs in and out of my room constantly; two pastors here to hold our hands and pray. The busyness made the day bearable. But now the silence was piercing. I felt so utterly alone: not merely in my room, but in the world.

The pain and isolation weren't so different, I imagined, from the immediate feelings of betrayal and despair in the moments after a lover has just walked out, leaving you for another. The lover who promised it was forever. The lover who was, and always will be, a part of you. The lover whose leaving takes away your will to go on for even one more day. The lover whose absence is felt so intensely that you believe your chance for ever finding happiness again is shattered forever.

How can anyone know what I'm feeling? Nobody…but Rachel! Rachel knew. When Rachel lost Sean, Alex was nine months old. I understood the love and attachment for a newborn, but couldn't fathom how that applied to a dead baby. And she took pictures with him! *How bizarre,* I remember thinking. When it happened, I reasoned that calling and asking about Sean might upset her, so I simply sent a card.

One month later, when Jeff and Rachel came home for Christmas, I sat visiting with Rachel, another cousin, and a sister-in-law. We were talking about babies and childbirth, and the conversation led to Sean. Rachel stopped mid-sentence, remembering I was three months pregnant. "I'm sorry Monica, I shouldn't be talking about this. I don't want to scare you."

"It's okay Rachel. I want to hear about Sean." *Besides, that wouldn't happen to me,* I thought to myself—

Now I understood too well, pictures and all.

And now it was too late in the night to call Iowa. I needed to talk to Rachel. Why hadn't she called me? Did she know I shared her fate?

I sighed and looked up at the clock. In the last forty hours, I had gotten less than two hours of sleep and knew I should be tired, but my mind raced. I looked over to my nightstand at the booklet from Candy. It had been staring at me all day, but I ignored it, knowing it would force me to face the reality of what had happened. Knowing it would make me cry. I gave in and picked up the book.

"Although it is normal to want to run away from much of what is happening to you right now, later you will be glad you chose instead to deal directly with your situation, even to the point of treasuring and gathering memories of your child's birth and death days." My eyes burned as I read, being reminded that I was still her mother.

Exhausted, I turned out the light welcoming the peace of unconsciousness, but sleep wouldn't come and I lay awake staring at the ceiling. I felt so alone, desperately missing Al. *Why didn't I ask him to stay with me tonight?* Always the martyr, I thought of Alex before myself, but I needed him more than Alex did right now. She had four grandparents to take care of her, and as far as she was concerned, this was one big family party. I wanted to call, but couldn't bring myself to wake him and tell him how stupid I had been.

I was still awake clutching wet tissues in my hand when light from the hallway suddenly poured into my room. "Are you having trouble sleeping?" said the faceless shadow. I nodded. The nurse left for a moment and came back with a sleeping pill. I knew she was trying to help, but a pill wasn't what I needed. *What I need is someone to hold me, tell me I'm not alone and that I'm going to get through this.* I took the pill from her and swallowed it, hoping to wipe out everything until morning when Al would be back. She disappeared into the bright hallway, shutting the door behind her and leaving me in the dark. I waited for the drug to do its wonder, but instead found myself waking every few minutes, my body so heavy I was unable to move, like a nightmare in which I was being chased by death itself, trying frantically to escape, feeling like I was running in a pool of molasses. It was another long night.

~ ~ ~

The first time I met Dr. Ross, I was instantly struck by his gentleness, subtle humor, and his resemblance to two of my favorite actors—somewhat of a cross between Steve Guttenberg and a young Elliott Gould. When he walked into my room early the next morning, he was suddenly more than my caring, handsome, forty-something doctor. He had accompanied me through the darkest night of my life, and I sensed I would always feel a bond with him that I would never be able to put into words.

Knowing he wasn't on call and didn't have to be here, I wasn't sure he would come, but I shouldn't have been surprised to see him. Dr. Ross treated his patients more like family members. Just weeks before, he had called me at home unexpectedly. "Is everything alright?" he had asked.

"Yes, everything is fine. I'm just anxious to deliver this baby. Where are you?"

"In the Virgin Islands with my son."

"You called from the Virgin Islands to check on me?"

"My wife told me one of my patients called looking for me, but didn't leave her name. I was worried something might be wrong."

"No, it wasn't me, but thanks for checking."

"Alright. I'll be back soon. Call me if you go into labor."

"I promise. Enjoy the beaches." I hung up smiling, wondering how many other expectant mothers would get a long distance call that day from a caring doctor on an island.

Now I sat in a hospital bed wishing I had been the one making that call to Dr. Ross telling him to please come home and deliver my baby before the knot pulled too tight.

"How are you?" he asked, pulling up a chair next to my bed.

"I'm tired and want to go home." Physically, I was recovering as expected but still on a liquid diet waiting for my bowel sounds to return. He wanted me to stay here until Friday. I wasn't sure I could last two more nights, with or without Al.

He told me the pathologist examined Miranda externally, and upon closer probe of her umbilical cord, confirmed that her blood flow had stopped at the location of the knot.

"I can't understand how she got so tangled up and tied a knot."

"Remember, she had a very long cord."

I tried to make sense out of a senseless death, wanting to find a reason, something or someone I could blame. "Maybe I took too many prenatal vitamins, and that's what caused her cord to grow so long."

He gave me a sad grin. "Alex didn't have a long cord and you took prenatal vitamins during her pregnancy." *He's right. But I still need a reason.*

"Is Al coming soon?" he asked.

"Yes, and my parents, too."

"Okay, I'll be back tomorrow." He smiled a sympathetic smile, patted my leg and walked out.

It was shift change time on the maternity floor and a new nurse barged in before I had time to respond to her knock. With straight, shoulder-length black hair, she looked to be in her thirties. "Time to check vitals." She was quick on task and short on words. "Arm up. Deep breaths. Open your mouth. Stay still." Then she checked to make sure I was voiding the appropriate amount of urine.

She reminded me of my ninth grade English teacher, Mrs. Carter. The entire school body called her Sergeant Carter. She knew it, laughed at it, even reveled in it I think, barking orders out in her no-nonsense way: "Wilson—she called us by our last names—Chapter 4, page 52, read out loud."

"Good news, your bowel sounds are back to normal. That means you can start eating real food."

"Thank God." I had had enough broth, jello, and tea to make even a tray of hospital food look like the cover of Bon Appetit.

"I'll be back later," said Sergeant Carter, the nurse, who was much younger and prettier than Sergeant Carter, the English teacher.

As she walked out, a young anesthesiologist came in to remove the epidural pump that had been supplying me with nonstop pain relief. He worked silently and was finished in a few minutes. "Congratulations," he said on his way out the door. "Thank you!" I called out without thinking. He disappeared into the hall by the time the shock registered.

"Doesn't everyone know my baby died?" I questioned Candy on the phone, repressing the urge to scream. She apologized and explained that there was a card taped to the outside of my door—a drawing of a leaf with a teardrop under it. It was supposed to notify staff that I had lost my baby.

She wanted to know which doctor it was, but all I could do was describe the man who breezed in and out, never introducing himself.

It was later that day when an elderly woman wearing a salmon-colored volunteer jacket came in to give me holy communion. "Congratulations. Did you have a boy or a girl?" I sensed anger steaming from my parents, who were now sitting with me after sending Al to the cafeteria for a much-needed break, and whispered that it was okay, this had happened before. Now I was experienced in these matters and remained calm, having already rehearsed my response after the last disaster.

"A girl, but she was stillborn."

"Oh, I'm so sorry!" I expected her to hurry out of the room, but instead she looked at me with knowing and told me that she lost eight children before finally delivering a healthy, full-term baby. My eyes widened as I pondered how anyone could be so strong. "We just trusted in God and kept living our lives. We never gave up hope that if we were meant to have a living child, we would eventually have one." I thanked her for sharing her story and she wished me God's blessings. After she left, I wondered if this woman, whose name I didn't know and who had given me a shot of hope and courage to face the days ahead, had been sent by an angel.

As my parents sat by my side, I sat in emptiness, my soul aching for my baby. *They wished that they had made better use of the limited time they had…* Words from the grief booklet echoed in my mind. *Be her parent,* whispered the voice in my head. My dad squeezed my hand and I burst into tears.

"I really miss her. I didn't get to spend enough time with her."

"Why don't you call Candy?" he said. "This might be your last chance. We'll be here with you."

A few minutes after I hung up the phone, Candy came in and sat down next to my bed.

"I didn't think I was going to hold her anymore, we already said goodbye, but I miss her so much," I told her.

"I think what you're trying to tell me is that you want to hold Miranda again," she said.

I nodded my head.

"I know this is hard for you Monica, but I'm glad you're doing this. I don't think the funeral home has come for her yet, but I need to check," said Candy, leaving.

A few minutes later, she came in pushing a bassinet. Trembling, I watched the small round figure move towards me, wrapped in a receiving blanket and wearing a tiny white hat with a pink ball on top, just like the one Alex wore the day she was born. Candy warned me that Miranda was still cold, but would warm up a bit. She carefully picked her up, laid her in my arms and then slipped out of the room.

"Oh, my poor baby. Why couldn't you have held on a little longer?" I asked her, rocking back and forth. My mom and dad sat on each side of my bed, wrapping their arms around me and Miranda. "It hurts so much," I cried out loud.

My dad hugged me tighter. "I wish I could take the hurt away, but I can't, so I'll just cry with you," he said in my ear.

Questions raced through my mind. *What was it like for you at the end? Did you struggle, or did you quietly go to sleep and never wake up?* I strained to remember any unusual movement that day. Maybe she kicked and squirmed trying to tell me something was wrong. Maybe I laughed at her acrobatics and patted my belly. I couldn't bear to think about it any longer and forced the thoughts away.

Emotionally exhausted, I let out a sigh. I unwrapped the blanket, smiling at the sight of the pink gown with white bunnies and a white satin drawstring at the neck. Candy told me this gown, along with the baptismal smock, was made by women who volunteer their time to sew for critically ill or stillborn babies. Pulling the hat off, I smoothed my hand over her hair. Her deep red lips reminded me of a punk rocker. I slipped my finger in her palm and wrapped her tiny fingers around mine, noticing the red tips that color coordinated with her lips. "It looks like someone painted her nails," I said, smiling.

My parents took turns holding her, and Candy came in to check on us.

"I can't understand why Al doesn't want to hold the baby again," I told her.

"Al is very caring towards you. I think he feels that he has to be strong, and holding Miranda again would interfere with that." I nodded, finally understanding.

My mom handed Miranda to me one last time, and I bent down to kiss her, resting my lips on her forehead for a moment. *Goodbye precious baby.* "I love you," I whispered in her ear, grateful that I had spent more time with her. The funeral director would be coming to take her body to the crematorium, and as Candy wheeled the bassinet out of my room, my parents held me while we cried together.

Sergeant Carter, the nurse, poked her head in my room to say she was going home for the day. She had been in and out all day and was starting to grow on me.

"Will you be back tomorrow?"

"I will," she answered with a quick smile.

~ ~ ~

Early Thursday morning, I sat alone in my bed wondering how my charmed life had been allowed to fall apart. Memories of childhood came flooding back: summer days filled with stick ball, Lake Michigan beach days along the Indiana Dunes, games of Marco Polo in backyard pools; winter nights of sledding, skating, neighborhood snowball fights.

An old boyfriend used to call my family the Brady Bunch. "Marsha Brady" was a grown-up 27-year-old now and had a husband, a house, and a happy, healthy two-year-old. Tragedy was something that happened to other people, people you read about in the paper or see on the evening news—not to Marsha Brady.

I had it all planned out: three kids, each spaced two years apart, at least one boy and one girl, preferably born in different seasons— spring, summer, and fall would be best. *This isn't how it was supposed to be.*

But now the dread of seeing or hearing newborn babies kept me secluded in my room when I was supposed to be up walking around. When Sergeant Carter, the nurse, walked in, I wondered if she would march me up and down the hall for drill practice. "Time to check vitals." *Here we go again.* "Arm up. Deep breaths. Open your mouth. Stay still." Then she did something unexpected. She sat down. To talk. Maybe I had broken barrack rules: too many visitors in my room; exceeding the phone call limit; a wrinkle in my hospital gown.

"How are you doing?" she asked. *How am I doing? Don't you mean, "Are you voiding?"* I thought to myself.

"I'm okay, I guess, just anxious to go home," I answered.

"Were you able to make funeral arrangements for the baby?" I told her our plans.

"And will you have support at home?"

"Yes, my husband, and my parents will stay with me for a while."

I knew these were routine questions—she probably had a checklist hidden under her clipboard—but her voice had softened, her tone sincere, and I couldn't be sure, but I thought I detected a hint of compassion, empathy even. "Sarg" had a heart.

When she got up to leave, I asked her to please page Dr. Ross and ask him if he would discharge me today.

"I will," she promised.

~ ~ ~

Candy was sitting by my bed when there was an abrupt knock and my door swung open. "So I heard someone wants to go home today," said a doctor strolling in with his nose in my chart, not bothering to introduce himself. I didn't recognize him, but since I hadn't heard from Dr. Ross and was ready to go home, I didn't care if he was Elvis.

He sat down to write my discharge order. "If it hasn't already, your milk should be coming in soon, in case you're planning to breastfeed." I looked at Candy with horror. *Sure, I'd love to breastfeed my baby if she wasn't dead!* I wanted to scream.

Candy was furious, but remained calm and laid her hand on my knee. "She's had a loss," she quietly informed the doctor.

He looked up, embarrassed, and quickly apologized. I said nothing. I just wanted to go home. He wrote me a prescription for painkillers, told me to go to Dr. Ross's office on Monday to have the staples taken out of my incision, and left.

"I'm so sorry Monica. There is no excuse for what just happened," said Candy.

"Doesn't he know what the card on the door means?"

"He should, but he probably didn't see it."

"How could he? He had his nose buried in my chart!" But why didn't he see it in my chart? *Maybe if the words "DEAD BABY" were plastered on the front of my chart, this wouldn't keep happening.*

When Al came to get me, Candy hugged us both goodbye, gave us her extension, and told us to call her if we needed to talk. I was going to miss her quiet empathy and reassuring smile.

~ ~ ~

I stepped out of my private shower, and Al wrapped me in a towel as Dr. Ross walked into my room. He was disappointed when I told him I had already been discharged by another doctor. "I'm sorry I didn't get here sooner, but I promised my daughter I would be at her ball game."

"I understand. I just have to get out of here." I was overcome by emotion, suddenly reluctant to leave. The moment I walked out that door, my pregnancy and all that went with it—eating for two, breast-feeding books, prenatal visits, planning and dreaming—would officially be left behind, and then what would become of me? It was as if I was hanging from the edge of a cliff by my fingertips, terrified to let go, not knowing how deep the hole was that I was about to plummet into.

"Can I have a hug?" I asked him. He wrapped his arms around me, and we stood for a moment. When I let go, he gently took my elbow and helped me over to the bed.

He pulled up a chair, sat down, and asked if we had any questions. I looked up at Al, who was standing beside me, and then back at Dr. Ross. "We'd like to try to get pregnant again. How long do we have to wait?" Somehow, amidst the chaos and turmoil, Al and I had discussed this already. Instinctively, we knew we could never replace Miranda with another baby—she would always hold a place in our hearts, an unfillable void—but we were so ready for another child and desperately needed something to hope for.

"You can try as soon as you feel ready."

"Physically or emotionally?"

"Both."

He asked if we knew about the Share support group Pat Vaci facilitated. We told him we did and were planning on going next month.

"The doctor who discharged me told me to come to your office on Monday to have my staples removed."

Dr. Ross shook his head. "No. I'll come to your house and remove the staples myself. You don't need to be sitting in a waiting room full of pregnant women." He wrote down my address and phone number and said he would see me on Monday. As he walked out the door, I nodded my head smiling, with a tear of gratitude in my eye, knowing that he lived thirty minutes away and was still on vacation.

~ ~ ~

After Sergeant Carter reviewed my discharge instructions, she was almost to the door when she stopped and turned around. "I don't know exactly what you're going through, but I do know what it's like to suddenly lose someone you love." *She's full of surprises,* I thought. The dozens of nurses and techs who had come and gone during my hospital stay had all been nice, but most of them treated me like I was another new mom because they didn't know what else to do or say. They came in, did their work, and left. Only a few had asked about Miranda or how I was doing emotionally; none shared anything about their lives.

"Will you tell me about it?"

She walked back over to my bed and sat down. One morning a short time ago, she woke up and found her husband lying next to her, dead. They never found the cause of his death, and now she was raising two young boys on her own.

"I'm so sorry, I didn't know." I reached over and put my arms around her. "You of all people know what I'm going through," I told her, and we talked for a long time.

I couldn't call her Sergeant Carter anymore; the name no longer seemed to fit. Her name was Carla, and I learned that she was a nursery nurse, but for some reason was pulling duty on the postpartum floor during my stay. Perhaps the universe had brought us together to share our stories and heal our grief a little bit more.

By the end of the ninth grade, Sergeant Carter, the English teacher, had risen to the rank of my favorite faculty member. By the end of my hospital stay, Sergeant Carter, the nurse, had achieved no less.

When I was ready to go, Carla came in with a wheelchair and informed me it was hospital policy. I was capable of walking and didn't want any attention drawn to me all the way out of the hospital, but let her help me down into the chair without objecting.

As we passed through the main doors of the maternity floor, two nursing managers sitting at a table doing paperwork looked up and smiled sympathetically. "Thank you for taking such good care of me," I told them.

"Thank you for being such a good patient," one called out as we got onto the elevator.

Carla saw the puzzled look on my face and smiled.

"Why did she thank *me*?" I asked.

"A lot of our patients are rude or demanding and don't want to cooperate when it's time to take vitals or draw blood. You were always so nice whenever we came into your room for something that we couldn't believe you had lost your baby."

I tried to imagine what it was like for a nurse, especially a young one, as she walked down the long deserted hallway to the isolated room at the end, wondering what lay beyond the door. Perhaps she might pause outside the room to catch her breath, gather her courage, and strain for any sign of what she was about to encounter. Would she find an inconsolable woman crying desperately for her baby? Or maybe a scene from the movie *The Exorcist:* eyes glaring, obscenities flying, and an order to "Get out!"

As Carla wheeled me through the main lobby, memories of leaving the hospital holding Alex came rushing back. Suddenly my arms felt so empty, and I hugged the manila envelope to my chest. Inside was all I had to show for a nine-month pregnancy, a baby who never took a breath, and dreams that would never come true: the pink gown with the white bunnies that Candy had removed from Miranda's body; the white cap with the pink ball on top; one receiving blanket. *How ironic: the moms going home with their babies don't get to keep the hospital receiving blankets; I get the blanket, but no baby.* Also inside: a souvenir birth certificate—*because she doesn't get a real one*—her footprints gently pressed on the back in ink; the name card from her bassinet that says I'M A GIRL! listing her birth information; her hospital bracelet; the white baptismal smock. Perhaps the most precious of the envelope's contents was a lock of Miranda's hair Candy had snipped and tucked inside a small, white envelope.

As strangers looked at me, I wondered if they could tell I had just had a baby. I felt so cheated; this was supposed to be a happy time. Instead, I was looking straight ahead, avoiding eye contact with anyone, trying to hold my emotions intact.

As Al pulled the car up, Carla gave me a hug, and we wished each other good luck. I slowly eased into the front seat, wearing the maternity outfit I had arrived in, and as we pulled away, I stared out the window looking for the world I had left behind just days before—the world I had known, and loved, and trusted.

6

Just over six weeks postpartum, I sit in the waiting room of Dr. Ross's office trying to ignore the new moms with baby carriers and pregnant women who walk in and out like models down the runway in a maternity fashion show. A few days ago, I realized my closet was still full of maternity clothes I was forcing myself to wear every day. I was hoping to fit into my regular clothes soon and didn't want to spend money on larger outfits. But the maternity clothes were a constant reminder of Miranda and my pregnancy, and I finally gave myself permission to go shopping. Determined to get into shape, I splurged on a new pair of walking shoes, too. I've been taking daily walks alone in a nearby wooded neighborhood, appreciating the sounds and smells of nature. Little by little, the fresh air and solace seem to be helping my soul to heal as well as my body.

Shopping, walking, I do anything to get out. I can't stand being in the house that should be echoing with the sounds of crying and cooing, giggling and gurgling; to look at the empty place where the bassinet should be rocking, or where the baby swing should be swaying; in a house where two children belong.

Everybody tells me it will take time. *Time, time, time.* I have more time than I can fill, and the hours and days are dragging. Can't I just fast forward through to the next year? Surely, someone has developed the technology. How much more time is it going to take before I will be happy again? Is happiness even available to me?

If only I can get through the next six weeks, I'll feel better physically, I told myself in the beginning. If only I can hang in there until I get my period back, we can try again. If only I can make it through a few more months, I'm sure to be pregnant and can really get on with my life. *If only…*

Just as a newborn starts to cry, Dr. Ross rides into the waiting room on a dashing black stallion, swings me up into his saddle and rescues me away from evil pregnant women who have surrounded me with their huge bellies. Okay, he doesn't have a horse, but he does come out and give me a hug, then quickly ushers me into an exam room, performing yet another chivalrous deed to protect me from unnecessary pain, second only to last month's house call to remove my staples.

After the exam, he tells me my uterus is back to its pre-pregnancy size and my incision has healed nicely. Then he pulls up his stool and sits down.

"How are you?" he asks.

"I'm doing okay. I have a lot of support, and I met Pat and made some new friends at the support group meeting."

He smiles and nods. "Any questions, concerns, complaints?"

"Shouldn't I be getting my period soon?"

"Well, most women typically get their period between six and eight weeks postpartum. Give it a few more weeks. If you still haven't gotten your period, then call me and we'll see what we can do to help it along." He gets up and walks towards the door, stops, and turns around. "Are you still moving to Houston?"

"I don't know. It's been put on hold for now." Al had accepted a job in Houston, and we were planning to move in the fall. I embraced the opportunity, looked upon it as an adventure. The grief booklet said to put off major decisions for at least a year—like job changes and moving. We were planning both. In our defense, the decisions were made long before the baby died, but alone in an unfamiliar city one thousand miles away from home, I would lose my entire support system.

A few weeks ago, Al got a call saying the Mexican economy was hurting, which was affecting the Texas economy, and the company that had offered him a job didn't know when, if at all, they could afford to pay another salary. The *For Sale* sign in the front yard came down, and I've started to wonder if perhaps the universe is shaking its head no to Houston. But part of me wants to flee to Houston now, leave the sadness behind, start over in a new city, in a new house, with a new baby…

"Well, for selfish reasons, I'm glad," he says. "I want to be the one to deliver your next baby." He smiles and walks out.

On the drive home from the doctor's office, I pass two grocery stores before I force myself to stop at the third, and last, store before I get home.

Alex begs for candy as I push my shopping cart into the checkout lane. My cart is filled with Hamburger Helper, frozen pizza, and Fruit Loops. That's about all I can manage for meals these days. Nobody is complaining. It wouldn't matter if they did. At least I'm at the store. For about a month, Al would call on his way home, and the conversation went something like this:

"Do you need anything from the store?"

"I don't know."

"Should I stop?"

"If you want to. I guess so. It doesn't really matter."

"What do you want me to do?"

"I suppose you could get some milk."

As I unload my groceries, a middle-aged woman pulls in line behind me. "Is she your only one?" she asks, smiling at Alex. Sometimes the question is, "How many children do you have?" Both haunt me since Miranda's death. These casual questions from curious strangers, once appreciated, now cause turmoil. Does a stranger really want to know that I have two daughters, but one is dead? The woman at the fabric store didn't.

It had been a beautiful, sunny day, and I was feeling unusually strong, independent, inspired—mostly nonexistent qualities since Miranda's death. I had taken Alex with me to buy materials to make a keepsake box for Miranda's things. I wondered what I would say to the clerk if she asked what I was making. Unsure of how people, especially strangers, would react, I decided to be vague and not mention my dead baby. While the clerk was measuring the lace I picked out, she asked if I was making something special. "Yes. It's for my baby." The woman smiled and nodded. "She died," I blurted out. The clerk glanced up with wide eyes, finished cutting, and quickly handed me the lace, not saying a word. I was horrified at what I had said and by what she hadn't said. I grabbed the lace in one hand, Alex in the other, and got out of there as fast as I could.

After that incident, I developed a plan of defense, deciding that if the person asking was a stranger in passing, I wouldn't acknowledge Miranda, which never failed to strike me with guilt, but I believed in the long run would save me from more grief. On the other hand, if the person was a new friend or someone I would see again, I would take a chance and share with them the fact that I had another daughter, but she was stillborn. The truth always felt better, and I almost always received compassionate responses. Today, I opt for the safe way out.

"Yes, she's my only one," I politely answer to the woman behind me and continue unloading my groceries, which now include a bag of M&Ms.

~ ~ ~

Two weeks later, Alex plays on the living room floor next to me as I sit staring out the window. *Is this how Katey Sagal felt?* I wonder, remembering the stillbirth of her daughter, Ruby, four years earlier. The actress who played Peg Bundy on the TV show *Married…With Children,* was eight months into her real-life pregnancy that was being mirrored by Peg's TV pregnancy. I remember the shock, the news stories, how the network wrote the pregnancy off as a bad dream. I wish somebody would rewrite my story, wake me up, and tell me it's all a bad dream.

It's been two months since losing Miranda. I strain to see her face, but it's hazy. Her life feels like a distant dream. *Did she exist? What did she look like?* Before I know it, I'm on my closet floor with Miranda's box in my lap, her pink bunny gown pressed against my cheek, tears falling. I close my eyes and am transported back to the hospital holding her in my arms. Inhaling deeply, I try desperately to detect any sign of new baby scent, but pick up only the smells of the box. I hold her blanket close, rocking, sobbing. *No, no! Why did you leave me? I miss you so much!*

Questions flood through my mind that I've held at bay for so long. *Where did you go? Was someone there to meet you, or were you all alone? Was it dark? Were you glad to go, or did you cry in grief, being torn from the comfort and safety of my body, your home for nine months?* All I can do is cling to my faith, believing she's somewhere, surrounded by love, light, peace. I can't allow myself to think anything else because the pain of it will destroy me.

I catch my breath and slide her photos out of the white quilted pouch with pink satin trim hand sewn for me by Rachel. My hands are shaking as I pull them out for the first time since getting them from Pat. She's more beautiful than I remember, but the redness of her cheeks and lips are a painful reminder, and I cry harder than I have since her memorial service. In the pictures, Miranda is lying in a bassinet surrounded by a stuffed teddy bear and a bunny, and in some, a lamb is cradled in her arm. She looks so sweet, I can't help but smile. *My baby. You were real. I touched and held you.*

I shuffle through her pictures, and after a few minutes a peaceful calm comes over me. As long as I have these pictures, I will never forget her face. As long as I hold and touch her things, I can feel close to her. She wasn't a dream.

"Mommy, Mommy," I hear from down the hall. I put the lid on the box and wrap the lace around it, finishing with a bow. Dad has the Polaroids, Al's brother has the ashes, and this is what's left of my baby, all wrapped up and placed neatly in an 11"x 18"x 6" box covered in floral contact paper. I force Miranda out of my mind and put the box up on a shelf, wiping my face so Alex won't see me sad, although I wonder if I'm doing her a favor by protecting her from my humanness.

Everyone thinks I'm doing great because they don't see me cry. "I don't think I could be so strong," they tell me one by one. They don't see me cry because I gain strength from their presence. My moments of despair, of complete breakdown, come when I'm alone. Even when I was a kid, I did my crying alone in my room. Now, instead of my room, it's my closet. I'm a closet crier.

Despite the love of my support system, I spend most hours feeling isolated in a world full of people who can't imagine what it must be like to be the parent of a dead baby. At the moment, I can think of few events more painful than the death of a child, and all other disappointments and irritations I've ever experienced, the ones I notice people all around me complaining about, are totally meaningless. As people around me engage in casual chit chat, I find myself walking away. All I want to talk about is life and death and the meaning of it all. As my circle of old friends grows smaller, a place in my heart makes room for the new friends who have found themselves in my life.

7

"You can stay home," I tell Al when this month's support group meeting comes around. I don't need his support there now that I have Dawn, Heidi, Beth, and Darlene to lean on.

"Are you sure?" he asks, trying to look concerned for me, but obviously relieved for himself.

"Yeah," I laugh, surprised to find myself looking forward to the meeting tonight.

~ ~ ~

I grab a seat next to Beth and Heidi, and we begin with introductions, which, I discover after my turn, I'm getting proficient at. As I sit listening to the anguish of a newly bereaved mother, an image flashes in my mind. I'm walking across a barren field, a red sky blazing overhead, an endless line of people stretching to my left and my right. As I turn to look behind, I see rows of men and women as far back as my eyes can reach. We march forward like soldiers, dropping one by one, yet the group goes on never looking back. This is how I feel about life lately. I'm muddling along, going through the motions, never knowing when it will be my turn to drop dead, or when I will suddenly lose another loved one. I shudder and force my attention back to the meeting.

It's Darlene's turn; I watch her closely. She's doing better this month. Beth told me Darlene has been spending time with her and Heidi during the long days.

Pat announces open sharing time. "David started school last month," says Heidi. "Brittany was due in August and I imagined taking him to school, pushing my brand new baby in the stroller. I dropped him off the first day of kindergarten, pulled the car over a block away from the school, and sobbed. It's really hard on David. He's asking if he's still a brother, why we didn't let him hold her, saying he wants to see her."

"I keep finding myself sitting in the rocking chair at night in the baby's room," I tell everyone, "thinking about Miranda and singing a lullaby I used to sing to Alex when she was a baby. *Hush a bye, don't you cry, go to sleep my little baby…*"

Heads nod.

After a few others share what's on their minds, a new mother asks if it's okay to send birth announcements. "I bought some for Joshua from a religious bookstore," says Beth. "After sending them to friends and family, Jeff and I finally got some acknowledgement and support—cards, flowers, special notes. But I also needed physical support like meals and visits. The grieving rituals in this country are so lacking. People don't know how to support someone who's grieving."

"Other cultures celebrate death as a passage into a better life," I say. "We, on the other hand, treat death as something unnatural, something to fear. And then when someone dies, we're encouraged by society to hide our feelings and get on with our lives. It's all so backwards. It's no wonder we're all struggling."

As the group shares a quiet moment, I realize my quiet habit has evolved from floor staring at the first meeting, to fidgeting with a damp tissue at the second meeting, and now I can look from face to face wondering who will speak next.

"I just quit my job here in Labor and Delivery," says Dawn. "I used to love my job, but lately it's gotten really hard. Multiple births are becoming more common. One day, my coworkers were raving about twenty-six-week-old twins saying, 'You should see their tiny little feet. You should see how cute they are!' *I don't want to see how tiny their feet are. Shut up and leave me alone!* I wanted to scream. Lately, I've been hearing about twenty-three-week-old babies doing fine. Why are they able to save other babies when they couldn't save mine?"

"Now that I'm not working, I spend more time at the cemetery," she continues. "I became friends with a woman whose daughter died of Leukemia five days before her sixteenth birthday and is buried near the triplets. We joked that her daughter, Andrea, was babysitting for my kids. I fill her angel birdfeeder for her, and she leaves surprises on the triplets' grave. I'll never forget something she said to me one day: 'It doesn't matter what age your child is when they die, it's tragic for all of us. It's no more tragic for me than it is for you. When a child loses parents, he's an orphan. When a woman loses a spouse, she's a widow. But there's no word for a person who loses a child. That's how awful it is. We're all equally in pain.'"

"After losing Nathan and Nicholas, I tried to go back to work when my maternity leave was up," says Darlene, "but I couldn't be around the same people I was with before—I didn't want to do anything I did before I was pregnant—and I quit after two weeks. I had to be around babies, I wanted to take care of something, so last month I got a job as a nanny for a ten-year-old girl and a one-year-old boy. The hiring manager knew I lost twins, and somehow I got through the interview without looking like a crazed mother who might steal someone's kids." Darlene laughs for the first time, and everyone joins in with her.

"Monica, last month you were talking about going back to work. Did you?" asks Beth.

"Yes, I did. It's been a good distraction, and I have a new friend who lost her dad and brother in a car accident, so we spend our lunch hour talking mostly about life and death and grief, but my interactions with other employees are so unpredictable. A woman in the bathroom told me how sorry she was and then as we were walking out, she added, 'Maybe it was for the best.'"

"Uh oh," says Heidi.

"Uh oh is right. I stopped and turned around to look at her. 'No. She was perfect and healthy. It was a senseless accident!' I told her. I know she meant well, but how can the death of any baby be for the best? Later, a woman from another department stopped me in the hall. 'You had your baby. Congratulations!' she said. *Oh God, not again. Doesn't anyone in this building know my baby died?* I thought to myself. This wasn't the first time I had been congratulated at work. She was embarrassed and felt horrible after I told her about Miranda. But she was nice and kept talking to me instead of rushing off with her tail between her legs. A woman passing by overheard me talking about the knot in Miranda's cord and suddenly stopped and said, 'When I was pregnant with my last one, we did an ultrasound a few weeks before my due date, and when the radiologist saw a knot in the baby's cord, they rushed me into surgery and did a c-section just in time to save the baby,' and then she breezed out the door. I felt like I had just been crushed by a giant boulder. I've been asking myself for three months if an ultrasound could have saved Miranda. I was angrier at that moment than when I opened a pregnancy book and read that it was impossible for an umbilical cord to have a knot."

After the meeting, a small group of us congregates in a huddle, sharing our ups and downs of the previous month while Pat makes her rounds talking to anyone who needs an ear or who lingers unsure of what they need. Thirty minutes later, Pat has her books packed up and is ready to lock up the room.

"I'm not ready to go home yet. Does anyone want to go to Omega?" asks Beth. Omega Restaurant, a Greek-owned family place, is a favorite among locals, offering everything under the sun from pancakes to pork roast, a bakery case that makes you want to skip dinner and move right on to dessert, and balloons for the kids. Everyone agrees, and one by one we pull out of the dark, empty parking lot in single file—Beth and Heidi, Dawn, Darlene, then me—like a midnight funeral procession.

~ ~ ~

Once seated around a large round table, Tony, a handsome dark-haired forty-something waiter comes to take our orders. "French toast," says Beth. "And a beer." Tony raises one eyebrow, I cringe, and everyone else laughs.

"What the heck," says Heidi, "I'll have what she's having. It's not like I'm pregnant."

"Me too," says Darlene. "It's not like I'm nursing a baby."

Tony, clearly amused, moves around the table one by one and finally stops at me. "I'll have French toast and orange juice." They give me that *don't be a sissy* look. "What? I don't even like beer!" I protest, and Tony winks at me as I hand him my menu.

"Do you remember our first meeting?" Beth asks. "Two months ago, I decided to go to that support group meeting with Heidi to help her out, thinking Heidi was such a basket case. But there I was bawling my eyes out with the rest of you, thinking *how are we ever going to smile again, how are we going to go on with our lives?*"

"And there was Dawn, having lost triplets, laughing with some friends," says Heidi.

"We all wanted to be like you," I say, pointing to Dawn.

Dawn tells us when she started coming to group the year before, everyone was newly grieving like her; there weren't any veterans who would come on a regular basis to offer support. So, as she rounded the corner of her first year, she continued going, not only for herself, but because of her need to let people know that they could get through this.

"I almost didn't come back to the second meeting," I confess. "The first one was so gut-wrenching."

"I tell people not to judge the group after the first meeting because it's going to drum up so many emotions, and you might be thinking *this is not going to help me,*" says Dawn. "If you can't go back right away, give yourself some time, but don't walk away after one meeting. Give it another try because each meeting gets a little easier. You'll make wonderful friends there that you can call anytime for support."

She tells us the story about a woman who came one night who had lost her baby a few years before on the same type of day, the same day of the week, and hadn't been to a meeting in a while. "I know you're probably thinking I'm supposed to be a good example, and here I am falling apart," the woman cried. "It's just one of those days. I knew I could come here and be safe. I knew I could come here and talk about it, and no one would judge me for it."

"It's really helped to talk to other women who have lost a baby," I say. "Before my first group meeting, I called two women I didn't even know after I found out they had lost babies."

"When I was collecting money for a March of Dimes Walk-a-Thon," says Dawn, "I met a neighbor who lost a baby the year before me. We became good friends and took walks together around the neighborhood. Sometimes it felt like people were looking at us saying, 'Look, there's the women with the dead babies. It's so nice they found each other. But don't talk to them, it might be contagious.' But we didn't care what people might be thinking. We helped each other get through bad days and knew we could say anything about our babies without being looked at strangely."

Like Dawn and her friend, Beth and Heidi have been relying on each other for solace and sanity, as well. Heidi tells us a story about a summer night not long after Brittany and Joshua died. It was about 1:00 in the morning, they met at a park, and Beth climbed into Heidi's car. Heidi had in her lap a box with roses on it, about the size of a shoebox. Beth's box was wooden. With Heidi's homemade lullaby tape playing on the cassette deck, they talked and cried and shared the contents of their boxes—photos and mementos of Brittany and Joshua—when suddenly the glare from a flashlight poured in on them through the driver's side window. The policeman leaned over and peered in.

"You're not supposed to be here ladies. The park is closed. Can I ask what you're doing?"

Beth looked at Heidi. Heidi looked at Beth, and then up at the shadowy figure. "Well, officer, both of our babies died and we're sitting here having a moment."

Silence.

"Um, okay ma'am, I'm so sorry, take as long as you need," he said and quickly left.

Everyone laughs.

"Can you imagine the look on his face?" I ask. "People don't know what they're getting into when they start a conversation with one of us."

Heidi tells us that she, Beth, and Darlene sometimes go to another support group at a nearby hospital to get an extra dose of help between our monthly meetings. But they all agree the format is regimented, with predetermined topics, and although it prevents people from getting stuck and talking about the same thing all night, the meetings end precisely at 9:00 p.m. and someone usually gets cut off in the middle of a sentence. "We've been telling people you can talk as long as you want at our Share group. I guess we're sort of recruiting," she chuckles.

Beth tells us they've also gone to a few support group meetings at the hospital where she delivered Joshua.

"So, they've become support group groupies," I say to Dawn, while grinning at Beth, Heidi, and Darlene as they laugh.

It's nearly midnight by the time Tony clears our breakfast plates and empty beer bottles, and we down the last drops of lukewarm coffee.

So begins a monthly ritual of French toast, beer—for those of us who can stomach it—and enough laughter to get us through another month until the next meeting. Unbeknownst to us, our round table at Omega will become a regular monthly event, and our group, which seems more like a club, will grow in membership.

~ ~ ~

As I drive home, I think about Beth who told us she's started babysitting at home for extra money, taking care of twin baby girls, five months old. I'm not sure if it's because she needs the money or because she needs to hold a baby. She also told us the monthly meetings aren't enough, and she's been seeing her counselor three times a week in addition to being on antidepressants. I know Beth tried going back to work after she lost Joshua and couldn't do it. But I can't help but wonder if this situation is helping her or adding to her stress.

Many of the women in our group planned to quit their jobs after the birth of their babies, and when their babies died, the women couldn't bring themselves to go back to work. Some of them have no living children to care for and sit home feeling lost.

"Monica, I'm glad you decided to go back to work," Pat said to me tonight after the meeting. "Sometimes you need another identity besides being a mother."

I knew she was right. Going back had been good for me. But the decision was one of the hardest I had ever faced.

8

I wondered how many friends I would still have at work. Eight weeks after delivering Miranda, my maternity leave was up, and my boss was expecting me back. When I was pregnant, I couldn't wait to quit my job. For nine months, I counted down with the help of a calculator:

80 more work days. I couldn't quit early because I needed the health insurance to pay for my delivery.

40 more work days. Then my department got sucked up by another one, my boss was leaving the company, and we were about to inherit a new boss who was known to be difficult.

20 more work days. I felt sorry for my coworkers.

10 more work days. This baby couldn't come soon enough.

Without a new baby, I no longer had my excuse to quit, and we still needed health insurance because the Houston move hadn't come through yet. But I liked the safety and security of being home with Alex and couldn't bear the thought of going to work now and sending her back to the babysitter. My coworkers wanted me back but, having young children themselves, understood and gave me the courage to make the call I had been putting off.

After getting bumped into my new boss's voice mail, I took a deep breath and spit out, "I'm really sorry, but I'm resigning because I can't come back to work right now. I'm really sorry." I hung up feeling like a coward, but relieved that it was over with.

A few minutes later my phone rang. It was my boss. She told me she hated to lose me, she knew this was a difficult time, and to stay home as long as I needed to. If I decided not to come back at all, she would understand, but if I decided to continue working, I could come back one day a week, two days a week, or whatever felt comfortable for me.

This was my second interaction with the new boss, the one who bites heads off and eats them for lunch, I had heard. The first encounter was in the hospital when she surprised me, walking into my room smiling sympathetically. When she gave me a big hug, sat down next to me and asked, "How are you?" laying her hand on mine, I held my breath, nearly in shock. She talked with the concern a parent has for her child, and later told me she has a young daughter. *Is this the same woman I've been warned about?* I wondered.

Her compassion on the phone caught me off guard, again, and I suddenly felt loyal to my new manager. *She really wants me, really needs me.* How could I not at least consider her offer? The extra time she offered took the pressure off so I could put work out of my mind for the rest of the summer. I told her I would come back in September and work two days a week.

Those extra weeks flew quickly, and before I had time to change my mind, it was Tuesday and I was due back at work. After hitting the snooze button on my clock three times, I finally dragged myself out of bed to start the morning routine. The thought of it made me sick. I had been enjoying time with Alex, and I knew she would rather be at home with me.

Why didn't I ask Dad to watch her, I wondered while driving to the sitter's house, remembering how Al's dad took care of Alex when she was almost one. Al's mom still worked, but his dad, newly retired and already bored, needed something important to do besides painting his garage walls and watching the Cubs lose. After five months, the two of them were buddies, and Grandpa was an expert on Huggies and Happy Meals. But I couldn't impose any longer—we needed Grandma and Grandpa on weekends, too—and finally settled on a babysitter. Her house was a mess, and instead of the cookie-baking granny type I was hoping for, she was more the pancake-flipping sergeant type. But at boot camp, Alex fit in with the kids and seemed to be happy.

Not today. I left Alex at the babysitter's house with her face pressed against the door crying "Mommy!" and pulled away quickly, wiping my stinging eyes with the back of my hand. *Damn it, why am I doing this? I'm sorry Alex, Mommy loves you, I'll be back soon. Please don't cry.*

Leaving Alex wasn't the only worry that plagued me. I was anxious about how my coworkers would react to me. Some, I knew, would be supportive, but I was returning to a newly merged department and a different manager, and I wondered who it would be most awkward for, them or me.

Once inside the building, I walked down the corridor to my putty-colored cubicle surrounded by putty-colored walls and dark carpet that looked like dirty putty when one of the vice presidents from another department stopped me. "Hi Monica, how's the new baby?" he asked with a big smile. I hadn't been here thirty seconds and already I wanted to turn and run for the door.

I forced a polite smile. "I guess you didn't hear. We lost the baby."

"Oh no, I'm sorry. What happened?" I told him about the cord accident and after he welcomed me back, I quickly headed for the safety of my cubicle.

My coworkers welcomed me back with hugs, and we sat talking for a long time. "I have something for you," said one of my friends handing me an envelope. "I wasn't sure if I should give this to you," she said apologetically. Inside was a photo of me taken at the going away party for our former boss. I'm smiling, happy as can be, and eight months pregnant.

"No, it's okay. It's the last picture I have of myself before I delivered Miranda. Thank you."

On the way down the hall to check in with my boss, I passed Carolyn, the secretary who sits across the hall from me. "Monica, you're back!" she said, her eyes lighting up.

"Thanks for coming to the memorial service," I told her, giving her a hug. We had become each other's cheerleaders during the past year. I encouraged her through college; she encouraged me through pregnancy. One week before Miranda died, she gave me a baby gift with a card that read *For the Baby-to-Be.* Inside she wrote, "Hope everything goes well and you have your beautiful little one soon."

Throughout the day, I was stopped by new coworkers, mostly women, several of them nurses, and welcomed back with compassion. *Maybe this won't be so bad,* I told myself.

I asked a friend how to find a woman named Lynne who had been on my mind ever since I received her letter in July.

July 7, 1995
Dear Monica,

I don't believe we have met yet; however, we spoke for quite awhile a couple of months ago when you interviewed me for the company newsletter. I remember our phone conversation well and have been looking forward to meeting you ever since. I am writing today to express my deepest sympathies to you and your family in the loss of your daughter, Miranda. It was only this last Friday that I learned of the tragedy that has come to you.

We spoke at length the day you called, but particularly about children and the excitement felt when expecting a new one to the family. I felt that maternal bond that comes from mothers/expectant mothers talking. Today I am writing because of another bond felt—that of experiencing tragic loss. Two years ago on July 2nd, my father and 16-year-old brother (13 years my junior) died in a weather-related car accident. It was unexpected and it was unwelcome, as is your loss, and although I have felt great pain and emptiness at no longer having them with me, I can only imagine the emptiness of losing a child—and I know I can never fully understand. In our department is a mom who lost her four-month-old child to SIDS. I did not know her at the time of her loss and although the losses and experiences are different, we can take comfort in each other; listening perhaps a little more closely, a little more appreciatively, than others who have not experienced sudden and tragic death.

I have no great words of wisdom and I fear all too few to comfort. One thing I have read and do know in my heart to be true—All life has purpose. Miranda's life within you had purpose, and I know she feels your love. I hope that we will meet, and I hope that we can talk and perhaps draw some small comfort from each other.

My thoughts and prayers are with you, your family, and especially with Miranda.

Lynne Schwartz

At the time of our phone interview, Lynne had two little girls and I was six months pregnant with Miranda, so our conversation had naturally turned to motherhood. I had hoped to meet her, but not under these circumstances.

I made my way through the maze of hallways and through a door. The woman behind the desk was close to my age, much younger than I expected for someone with her wisdom and compassion. "Lynne?"

"Yes."

"I'm Monica."

She jumped up and came around her desk. "I'm so glad to meet you," she said, wrapping her arms around me for a long moment.

"Me too."

If it hadn't been for her letter, I don't know if I would have gone back to work. We quickly became close friends, often spending our lunch hour together, sharing life stories and struggles with grief.

Lynne introduced me to the mother who lost her baby to SIDS, who gave me a card with a sketch of a child resting in the palm of a large hand, like the one on the cover of Miranda's memorial service program. Later, I learned that she and her husband were divorcing. My heart broke for her as I tried to contemplate the devastating loss of a child and a marriage in such a short time.

I also learned that one woman in my department had suffered three miscarriages and another had lost twins. Suddenly it was like I had been drafted onto a team, the tragedy team, and had support from teammates as I faced the days ahead in my cubicle in the isolated corner of the building.

Driving home, I realized I had made the right decision. My co-workers were more supportive than I hoped, allowing me to share Miranda's life with them. And I needed something else in my life to focus on besides missing my dead baby and conceiving a new one. The sitter told me Alex cried only until losing sight of my car and had been happily playing all day.

~ ~ ~

Now that I was earning a paycheck again, I had no financial excuse not to pay the medical bills that were piling up. The funeral home had waived its charges for picking up Miranda's body and arranging for her cremation. Somehow I expected that the fees for having a baby should also be waived if you didn't get to keep the baby. That little voice inside was screaming out at the injustice. I scanned the front and back of each statement looking for a payment option that read:

☐ **Decline payment due to unfair outcome and unbearable grief!**

Writing out the checks was like swallowing three bitter pills: $420 to the hospital, $108 to the anesthesiologist, and $445 to the physician's office, whose statement told me to *"Have a Nice Day!"*

My disappointment in having to pay medical bills was overshadowed by having to pull out the tampons. Sometime during the summer, my period had resumed and I was hoping it would be short-lived. *I waited forty-one days for this?!*

9

Although physically I'm back to normal, my emotional state is a teeter-totter ride. I still can't handle being alone during the day and wonder if I'll ever be able to stay home by myself like a big girl. Alex won't go to sleep at night without one of us lying on the floor next to her toddler bed, and I can't help but wonder if my fear of being alone has radiated to her.

For temporary relief on a weekday afternoon, Al has taken Alex and me to the shopping mall to get us out of the house. We sit on a bench eating ice cream cones, marveling at Alex's excitement at throwing pennies into the fountain. It's her favorite thing to do here, and we're not allowed to leave until all pennies have been scavenged from purse and pockets and thrown wildly into the water.

I notice every pregnant woman who walks by, and feelings of jealousy flood through me. It's more than protruding bellies I envy. I look at their faces and see naïve happiness, joyful expectations, still-on-the-fairy-tale-side-of-pregnancy dreams: baby showers, pickles and ice cream, storks and happy homecomings. *That used to be me.*

I look the other way. *Here comes another one.* She's young, no kids tagging along. *This must be her first.* Carrying bags from the maternity and baby stores, looking as if her biggest worry is whether she should be buying pink or blue, she's the epitome of pregnant innocence. I long for that feeling. But pregnancy will never be this way for me again. *So why should it be for anyone else?* I plead.

I run up to her and scream, "Don't you know your baby could die, like mine did? Don't look so happy. You're not out of the woods yet! And, for God's sake, don't buy any baby clothes until you know the baby is coming home alive!"

I don't really do it, wouldn't really want to, would be horrified if I did. But these thoughts creep into my mind, and I don't know what to do with them. Tragedy has introduced me to a cynical part of myself that I've never met before.

Unfortunately, it doesn't stop there. The death of my baby has wrapped me in a thick layer of fear and vulnerability about life, which probably explains why I can't stay home alone. If my baby could die in the blink of an eye, so could my two-year-old. I'm haunted with visions of her being taken by a stranger, or falling to her death on the playground, and keep her within arm's reach wherever we go, strapped, buckled, or otherwise attached.

An unexpected card in the mail tells me I'm not the only one still struggling. *For every tear that falls from your eyes…there's a prayer in my heart for you,* it reads. I suddenly feel as sad as the teddy bear on the cover looks and quickly open the card.

> *Dear Moni,*
>
> *I've had this card for you for awhile now, but I still have a hard time doing anything tangible concerning Miranda. I guess because it makes it more real and as you know, I'm not doing too well with losing her. But now, my thoughts are with you. I want to be there for you in any way I can. I'm here for you to lean on. I hope you know how very special you are to me! You're in my thoughts every day.*
> *I love you so much,*
> *Your mom*

I close the card sobbing, remembering how my mother took care of me after Miranda died. After staying with us for six days during and after my hospital stay, my parents, both due back at work, packed for their return to Indiana. My mom must have sensed my terror at the prospect of being alone. "Do you want me to stay for a few more days?" she asked, coming to my rescue with a mother's intuition.

My eyes lit up. "Could you?"

"There's no place else I'd rather be," she said.

"What about work?" I asked.

"I told them I don't know when I'll be back, and they told me to take as much time as I need."

"Thanks Mom," I whispered with a hug. Over the years I had convinced myself, like most girls, that I didn't need my mother anymore now that I was a grown-up. In truth, as independent as I had become, I still needed her very much.

But ever since then I've avoided talking to my mother about Miranda because I couldn't bear both her sadness and mine. It's difficult to fathom a grandparent's pain when a child dies: our parents grieving over the loss of a grandchild and hurting for their own children, yet trying to be strong for the family. Mom tried unsuccessfully to find a support group for grandparents near her home, and although she occasionally attended one for parents at a local hospital, she never felt she fit in.

I calm myself down and pick up the phone. I want to tell Mom how much I appreciate her card and how sorry I am that I haven't turned to her for support more often since Miranda's death. Maybe the pain has dulled just enough that we can lean on each other without completely losing it.

~ ~ ~

As the days go by, I seem to be making progress: less Hamburger Helper, more meatloaf. I've started enjoying my favorite things again, like curling up next to Al on the couch and laughing at *Seinfeld*.

But it takes only a moment to trigger those still-familiar feelings and it all comes rushing back. Baptisms at church, mothers with babies, families with two little girls: live pictures of what I'm missing.

Alex's loss of a little sister contributes to my sadness. I had always planned to have my children close in age, and every month that goes by pushes that dream further from my grasp. Alex loves babies so much, I have to watch closely that she doesn't smother them as she leans over them in their carriers for kisses and hugs. Taking care of her baby sister would have been a big deal to her, and although Alex doesn't know what she's missing, I do.

Getting my period back has given me something new to focus on. *You can't successfully say hello to your next baby until you have said good-bye to this baby…and saying goodbye takes time,* echoes words from the grieving booklet *When Hello Means Goodbye.* I know, I know, but I don't have too much sense these days, and the thought of another baby gives me enough hope to get through each day.

I got pregnant quickly with the first two, but I'm not leaving this to chance. A book tells me how to pinpoint ovulation and the best time to conceive. Every morning I take my basal body temperature before getting out of bed, waiting for the temperature shifts that might signal ovulation. Every afternoon, I stick my hand down between my legs and check for changes in my cervical mucus, waiting for the thin, clear, stretchy conditions that also signal ovulation. I write it all down on a chart.

"What's this?" Al asks when I return from shopping and drop a bag in front of him.

"Boxer shorts."

"Boxer shorts?"

"I read in a book that wearing boxers will keep your testicles cool, which will boost your sperm count, which will increase our chances of conception."

"Do I really have to do this?"

"Please?"

Sigh. "I guess I can try."

On my way out the door, I stop and turn. "Oh yeah, can you also stop drinking alcohol and stay out of hot tubs?"

"Oh, come on!"

"Just for a few months. Please?"

"That's supposed to help my sperm count?"

"Yep."

"Anything else?"

"Nope."

Sigh.

To cover all the bases, I buy an ovulation predictor kit. Spending twenty-five dollars for the kit is nothing to an obsessed woman on a mission. Every day for five days I have to aim my pee down between my legs onto the tip of a skinny stick. I finally figure out that it's easier to pee in a cup and pour the pee on the stick.

~ ~ ~

In lieu of a regular meeting this month, the hospital is holding a memorial service in the chapel. I feel I should be here for Miranda's sake, but am apprehensive, suspecting an overly emotional experience, especially if music is involved.

Pat is greeting families at the door. Al makes name tags for us, and I find the candle with Miranda's name on it. Inside, I set a picture of Miranda on a table next to the altar. My eyes scan the photos, keepsakes, or symbols of other babies who share the table with her. We find two seats together and sit down in the intimate candlelit chapel.

I turn around anxiously, looking for my friends. Beth and Heidi are behind me to the right sitting with their husbands, whom I have never met. Later, I find out Heidi's also dragged her in-laws here to sit and listen to her sob through the whole program. Dawn and Darlene, with their husbands Andy and Larry, whom I've met once or twice at meetings, are on the other side of me, along with many other couples I recognize from the past three months.

Sitting alone at the end of the room is Dr. Ross, wearing hospital scrubs, and I suddenly remember that Thursday is always his day on call. I wonder if he's here just for me, but I know he and Pat are close friends. Nevertheless, he is the only doctor here, and he's my doctor.

"Those who have not experienced the death of an infant or the loss of a pregnancy may not understand. Yet those of us here know these precious babies have touched our lives deeply," Pat opens. My thoughts wander to an image of holding Miranda close. Now I'm sitting alone in the closet crying into her blanket. I fight the tears back and force my attention back to Pat. "Love cannot be measured by the amount of time the child lived on this earth. And that love does not stop with death. Parents will never forget their child."

Heidi gets up and reads a poem she wrote. *She's brave.* She chokes up after the first line, and we all hold our breath silently urging her to hang in there and get through it.

Oh no, music. The musicians are playing "Be Not Afraid," a song I once enjoyed singing at church when I was younger. But when I was younger, I had no concept of the verse "blessed are you that weep and mourn, for one day you shall laugh." Now I understand. Too choked up to make a sound, I mouth the words and reach for one of many tissue boxes placed strategically throughout the room.

Each child's name is called, or if the child doesn't have a name, "baby" is substituted for the first name. "Miranda Blair Novak." I walk up to the front to receive a keepsake dove pin. We light our candles, passing flames from one parent to the next, saying our baby's name as our flame is lit.

When the musicians play "On Eagle's Wings,"—another once-favorite song that I can't manage to sing—the verse "He will hold you in the palm of His hand" reminds me of Miranda's memorial service cover. I'm relieved when it's over and take a deep breath, glancing over to see Dr. Ross talking with another couple. *So, I'm not his only patient with a dead baby.* Jealousy hits me at the thought of having to share him—which seems completely silly and irrational—but he soon walks over to shake Al's hand and give me a hug. "I'm surprised to see you here," I say.

"Well, I try to come when I can." His beeper suddenly goes off and he shakes his head. "I'm sorry. I have to go. It was good to see you both."

"Hopefully I'll see you soon for a prenatal visit," I tell him.

"I hope so too," he smiles.

Jealousy floods me again with the thought that he's going off to deliver someone else's live baby.

Out in the hall, we join the others for punch and cookies. "I didn't mean to ignore you all in there, but I knew if I looked at any of you, I'd lose it," I tell my friends. They laugh.

"We were all thinking the same thing," says Beth.

~ ~ ~

"You're quiet," says Al, looking over at me as I stare out the car window. "Are you okay?"

"Yeah. It's just that tonight's memorial service brings it all back, like it was yesterday. I know I've come a long way, and it doesn't hurt so often or as sharply as it did in the beginning, but the details of that first week, I don't think I'll ever forget."

10

The two days leading up to the memorial service were a blur except for a few all-too-clear moments. The first time I walked into the nursery the baby was going to share with Alex was one of these. It was Thursday, and we had been home only a short time from the hospital. I slowly climbed the stairs and stopped at the top to catch my breath. My parents had already dismantled the bassinet in my bedroom because they thought it would be too hard on me to see it, ready and waiting for a sleepy newborn. But I didn't know if the other baby things remained. Looking down the hall at the last door on the right, I wondered what I would find inside.

I was welcomed by Yippie Coyote in pale southwestern colors of orange, purple, and green, the theme we chose when I was pregnant with Alex. Diapers and blankets were stacked underneath the changing table exactly as I had left them. Sleepers and gowns neatly lined the two top dresser drawers, waiting to be worn. I was surprised to find that nothing had been touched.

Taking a deep breath, I pulled open one of the dresser drawers filled with underwear, pajamas, and booties. I lifted out the white velour sleeper Alex had worn—a gift from a college friend, it was my favorite—and pressed against my face the soft fabric that still smelled of baby-fresh Dreft.

I remembered the day just a few weeks earlier when Alex and I prepared for Miranda's homecoming. She had helped me clear out two of the drawers for the baby, eager to share her room and her dresser. What fun it had been washing, folding, and putting away tiny things as we talked about what it would be like to be a big sister, whether it was a boy or a girl, and the name we would choose.

She was supposed to be Samantha. The grief booklet said, "Allow your next child to be her own person. Choose a new name. Don't imply that the new child is a replacement for this dead child by 'saving' the old name. It rightly belongs to your dead child." But that's exactly what I had done: I'd saved the name for a new child, stealing it away from the dead one. Now I felt guilty and didn't think I could ever use the name Samantha.

Next, I opened the closet and was greeted by a dozen baby boy outfits, tags still attached, hanging in a row. What excitement when I'd discovered the huge clearance sale at the baby store, outfits marked down to two dollars. All that remained were boys' clothes, but certain I was having a boy, I grabbed one of each. When Al came home that day and saw the outfits spread out on our bed, the look of disbelief on his face was priceless. "But what if it's a girl?" he had said shaking his head.

Someday soon, I knew, I was going to have to deal with all of these little reminders in order to bring closure to Miranda's death. But right now I didn't want closure; I wanted my baby.

When I came out of the nursery, Al was waiting for me at the end of the hall and handed me a piece of paper.

"What's this?" He looked at me, but said nothing. "Why is Everyone So Sad?" was written across the top of the page in his neat printing. I glanced up at him for a moment, then continued reading.

Usually when I walk into a room, everyone calls my name
and wants to play.
Not today.
Everyone is sad.

Why is everyone so sad?
Did everyone get an "owie"?
Or maybe they have to go to bed early.
Now, that is sad.
Mommy is in a funny bed and will not hold me.
She's not talking very loud.
She's sad.

Why is everyone so sad?
I woke up today at Grandma & Grandpa's house.
That was nice, but why am I here?
They're sad.

Why is everyone so sad?
Daddy holds me extra tight and kisses me a lot.
His tears fall into my hair.
He is sad.
Why is everyone so sad?
Mommy's tummy is not big anymore.
Where's the baby she said was in there?

Now I'm sad.
I guess it's okay to be sad.

"You wrote this while I was in the hospital?" I asked him. He nodded. I pressed my face against his chest, his shirt soaking up my tears, and he wrapped his arms around me while we stood in silence.

~ ~ ~

That night Al and I lay in bed holding each other. It had been a long time since we could cuddle so closely without a bulging belly in the way; now I could lie comfortably in any position. And the irritating heartburn was gone. No longer would I have to trek downstairs at 10:00 p.m. for a glass of chocolate milk, my nightly indigestion cure. I slid my hand down over my stomach remembering those familiar movements. *Nothing.* Full of life just days before, now I was empty and still. "I miss her inside of me," I sobbed.

"I know," he whispered. It was too dark to see if he was crying too.

~ ~ ~

The next morning, Friday, as I walked into the kitchen where my parents were eating breakfast, I noticed two envelopes on the counter. The first one, from the crematorium, contained a receipt for $60 for the "cremation of Baby Miranda Blair Novak." I tried to imagine the feelings that ravaged Al as he wrote out the check to pay for the cremation of his baby girl's body.

My dad watched me from across the room as I picked up the second envelope, a large manila, and traced my fingers across his neatly printed words: PICTURES OF MIRANDA.

"You don't have to do this now," he said, looking concerned when I brought the envelope over to the table and sat down.

"I know. But I want to." That was a lie. It was something I had to do and was afraid I wouldn't have the courage after my parents went home.

"I need to tell you that some of the pictures might upset you," he said gently. I nodded my head to acknowledge his warning, slowly opened the envelope and pulled out the pictures, tears already rolling down my cheeks. I held a photo of my mother looking down at the baby gently cradled in her arms. I had never seen my mom so sad. Miranda looked just as I remembered with dark hair, brick-colored lips and red cheeks. I quickly flipped to the next picture. Dad's hand was resting on the baby's head, and Miranda's tiny white hand was wrapped around one of mom's fingers.

I turned to the next photo and suddenly felt like I had been kicked in the stomach. Miranda's clothes had been removed and she was lying on her back with her head turned to one side. This was the first I had seen her without a blanket or gown and was shocked by the dark, red marks covering her entire body, as if she had been severely beaten.

"Candy said the red areas are where the blood settled," Dad explained.

"I never want to see this picture again," I cried, shoving the photos back into the envelope. "Will you please take them home with you and keep them for me?"

"Sure, they'll be waiting for you when you're ready for them again." I wondered if that day would ever come.

"Did you know my sister Betty had a stillborn baby?" he asked.

"No," I answered, sniffling, astonished nobody had ever talked about it. "What happened?"

"It was a boy. She was about eight months along." My dad had no more information. Later, I asked my grandma about the baby. She told me my Aunt Betty was pregnant with her second child. It was the early 60s. She started hemorrhaging, they gave her a blood transfusion, but they couldn't save the baby. Then she had a miscarriage after that. She already had Patti and couldn't go through another pregnancy again. I always wondered why my cousin Patti was an only child. Grandma didn't know if Betty held the baby, named him, or even if he was buried; Aunt Betty never talked about it.

Mom and I took Alex outside to play, trying to keep the house quiet so Al could attempt to work. Still sore from surgery, I sat in a chair in the driveway watching my mom push Alex back and forth down the sidewalk in her Little Tikes minivan. My two-year-old provided a much-needed distraction from thoughts of tomorrow's memorial service.

One of my neighbors, an elderly widow and mother of eight grown children, walked over to talk to me. "I heard about your baby. I'm sorry."

"Thank you," I smiled up at her.

"You're young, you'll have another one." I nodded. She meant well, and a small part of me found comfort in her optimism. But what she didn't realize was at that moment, I didn't want another one. I wanted Miranda. No other baby could possibly take her place; ten babies would never fill the hole losing her had left in my life.

After being forced inside by a sudden rain shower, I felt drawn back outside. The sun was shining against a black eastern sky; a few remaining drops of rain fell on my face. *Where are you? Can you see me, hear me? Do you feel how much I love you, do you know how much I miss you?* whispered my heart. Feeling completely disconnected from my baby, I prayed she was in a safe place, peaceful and beautiful, surrounded by love. It was the only thought that made me feel even remotely better.

As I looked out toward the gloomy sky, a rainbow appeared, full and vibrant. I remembered reading long ago that in many cultures, the rainbow was believed to be a bridge between heaven and earth, sometimes seen as a message of hope, other times thought to be a path to the gods along which the souls of children were called. I marveled at its beauty when a second rainbow emerged, just above the first one. I couldn't remember the last time I had seen a double rainbow. It was incredible. A sudden warmth in my heart brought with it the undeniable feeling that this was a sign meant for me, from God or perhaps from Miranda, telling me she was okay, that she was still with me in spirit. It's what I wanted to believe. I watched and wondered until the rainbow faded away.

I sat down in the lawn chair alone with my thoughts. Moments later, a car pulled up in the driveway next door and drew me out of a daze. My neighbor, Thelma, babysat for a little girl, and the girl's mother had come to pick her up. Over the months, this woman and I had gotten to know each other and often talked about our kids, who sometimes played together.

"How are you feeling?" she asked, smiling, unable to see my significantly smaller belly under the oversized shirt I wore.

"Thelma didn't tell you?"

"Tell me what?"

"I lost the baby."

"Oh. I'm sorry," she said, frozen in her tracks, and then quickly disappeared into the house, never speaking to me again, except for a quick "hi" and "bye" on her way in and out each day. I was surprised and hurt that Miranda's death would make someone so uncomfortable she would withdraw from me. Trying to put the incident out of my mind, I went inside for the lasagna dinner that my former coworker Debbie had somehow prepared and delivered despite her full-time job at the office and her other full-time job as single mother of two.

~ ~ ~

At the church on Saturday morning, I stood in the hallway, trying to mentally suppress the pain from my incision and emotionally suppress the anxiety creeping into my heart. Earlier, I had functioned on autopilot, getting out of bed, showering, dressing in a flowing floral maternity dress, and eating breakfast without realizing it. The impending memorial service put knots in my stomach and made my hands shake.

Pastor Needham asked if we were ready to begin. We couldn't put it off and nodded with resignation. The church was full of family, old friends, new friends, and coworkers. Many had driven over an hour from Indiana. Rachel had driven six hours from Iowa. As we walked down the center aisle, all eyes upon us, I was suddenly transported to our wedding day. We were walking on clouds then, happy and full of hope. Now it took every ounce of strength I had to get down the aisle without falling apart.

We took our seats in the front pew, and my eyes locked onto a small table at the front of the altar. With the exception of the photos and lock of hair, which as far as I knew had been left at home, Miranda's mementos were carefully arranged for all to see: items from the manila envelope Candy gave me, plus a soft pink dolly from Grandma with a tag that read: *My First Doll.* It would be her only doll.

It was so important to me for everyone to see these things of hers that minutes before, I asked Pastor Needham to announce to everyone to please come up to the front at the conclusion of the service and take a look. He gently explained that those who wished to would do so on their own.

Why didn't we have a real funeral with a casket and a wake so everyone could see and touch her and know she was real? I argued with myself. *No, we made the right decision. You couldn't bear to put your baby in a box and bury her in the ground. Besides, we're moving to Houston and can't leave her behind,* I reminded the other half of myself.

I looked down at the program someone had handed me. On the cover was a sketch of a small child with her eyes closed, resting peacefully on the palm of a large hand. *I will not forget you. Behold, I have engraved you on the palms of my hands. Isaiah 45:15b-16.* I wondered if the church always used this cover for children that die, what few there were.

"The Lord is my shepherd, I shall not want. He makes me lie down in green pastures, he leads me beside quiet waters…though I walk through the valley of the shadow of death…" read the congregation while I forced the tears back. Never in my life would I have believed I would say these words for my own child. God, this is too much.

When Pastor Needham stood up to give his sermon, I wondered what he could possibly say to make sense out of any of this. What comfort could he bring us? How would he explain why God had allowed my baby to die? He gazed at us, then around the church, and began. "My wife and I were taking our evening walk and were greeted by our neighbor with the news of birth. 'It's a girl!' 'What great news!' The next morning, I got the call from Al asking me to come to the hospital. Their baby girl, Miranda, was stillborn. The irony was more than I could handle as I backed out of my driveway and saw the big plywood cut-out of a stork in our neighbor's yard—and I had to go to be with parents whose joy had been turned to sorrow.

"Monica, Al, we can only imagine—no, we can't even imagine—how deep your hurt and loss are, to carry a child to full term and to have to deliver it stillborn. Unless we experience it ourselves, we can never comprehend that pain.

"What we can do is care. What we can do is try to surround you with our love. What we can do is turn, together, to the One who promises to accompany us in our most painful moments." He said he refused to believe God chose to take our baby, that he couldn't serve a God who would do that to loving parents. Although he had no answers, I found satisfaction in his defense of God. If he had tried to tell me God had a reason for taking my child, I don't think I would have ever stepped foot in another church again.

At the end of the service, while the pianist played softly, Al and I stood, crying, and tried to muster the courage to walk out. Alex, wrapped in her daddy's arms, began to cry, unsure of what was happening, but knowing something was terribly wrong. As we turned and carried her towards the back of the church, I saw my aunt put her arms around my brother Brian who was sobbing.

Born only eighteen months apart, the close relationship I shared with Brian through the years was my inspiration for wanting to have my own children close in age. When he came to the hospital, he broke down crying and asked to see Miranda. I told him Candy had already gone home for the day, and I hated to inconvenience her. Never wanting to inconvenience anyone himself, my brother told me not to worry about it. But it would forever nag at me, knowing that spending one special moment with the niece he would never get to play checkers with or take to the park would have meant a great deal to my younger brother.

A few rows back was Aunt Judith, my mother's sister. She and my uncle came to the hospital the night before I went home. Family had gone and Al and I sat in my quiet room talking when a nurse came in to tell me they were out in the hall, raising her eyebrows as if to remind me that visiting hours were over.

"I didn't know she was coming," I said out loud, signaling my surprise to the nurse.

"I can tell them to come back tomorrow during visiting hours."

"No, it's alright, they can come in."

My aunt and uncle hugged us and asked how we were. Five minutes passed with no clues as to why they had shown up so late without warning.

"Can I hold Miranda?" my aunt asked. *So that's it. She came to hold my dead baby, but why?* Seeing my aunt approximately twice a year during holidays, her request was almost a shock.

"The only person that can bring her to me is Candy, and she's already gone for the day. I would have to page her to come in, and I don't even know if Miranda is still here."

"Oh," she answered, her disappointment evident.

A few minutes later they said goodbye and quickly left. Al and I looked at each other speechless.

I quickly dialed my mom. "Mom, Aunt Judith was just here and wanted to hold the baby. Why would she do that?"

"I don't know."

"Will you please call her and tell her I'm sorry she didn't get to hold Miranda, but she caught me off guard. It was late, I was upset and didn't know what to do."

My mom told me a few days later that my aunt had a miscarriage many years ago. She never dealt with the grief of losing her baby and thought maybe, by holding Miranda, she could somehow come to terms with her own loss.

My aunt still remembered vividly the day it happened, February 4th, 1967. She had recently given birth to her first son and found herself pregnant again soon after. She was excited that her two children would be exactly one year apart, just as she and her younger sister were. But when she miscarried the baby, her dreams fell apart and her husband told her to stop crying. Her family knew about the miscarriage, but they were in another state, and without any support, Aunt Judith held her grief in, still carrying it in her heart nearly thirty years later.

Now I understood. *If only I had known.*

I pulled my focus ahead to the back of the church, avoiding eye contact with anyone. Family and friends watched, waited, wiped their faces, and followed behind.

Downstairs, the funeral committee had a luncheon waiting. These people, most of whom I didn't know, had given up their Saturday morning to set up tables, prepare and serve food, and clean up. I ate, what little I could, and watched family and friends talking, laughing, hugging, Alex and the other kids chasing each other around the tables while, unbeknownst to me, my father was walking around showing photos of Miranda to anyone who cared to see.

Afterwards, I walked outside into the sunshine, and my baby brother Eric handed me a small white flower he had picked from the ground. At seventeen, Eric was hardly a baby, but I couldn't kick the phrase. I remembered the day my parents brought him home from the hospital and I held him for the first time, a bundle of wonder to a nine-year-old girl. Fifteen years later, when we brought Alex home from the hospital, Eric snatched her up and sank into the couch. Shortly later we found them both sound asleep, a new bundle of wonder in the arms of a giant teddy bear.

I gave him a hug and slid the flower into my purse, wondering what this young man, ready to take on the world, must be thinking with his sudden awareness of life's uncertainty and unfairness.

As we walked down the stairs and headed for our cars, I was unaware that Papa, my 89-year-old grandfather, had walked out behind me, sobbing uncontrollably. I had never seen Papa cry and I suppose he wanted to keep it that way.

Papa was a veteran of this thing called death. His mother died when he was six. He lived through the Great Depression, countless wars, and at his age, had buried enough family and friends to fill a cemetery; attending a funeral was a weekly event for him, yet here he was sobbing for a little baby girl he'd never laid eyes on.

At home, neighbors carried in baskets of flowers delivered in our absence, and a woman from the church altar guild brought the flowers that had decorated the sanctuary during Miranda's service. When I had first come home from the hospital a few days earlier, I'd hardly recognized my living room transformed into a floral shop by flower baskets and plant arrangements from friends, cousins, coworkers, even Al's business acquaintances. Now my floral shop had grown into a botanical garden.

Brian turned on the stereo and put on one of my favorite CDs. A week earlier, I was listening to this, dancing around the house with Alex. But now, a good beat was like fingernails on a chalkboard, and halfway into the first song I turned it off.

I headed for the freezer, pulled out two large cabbage leaves and tucked them inside my bra. Candy, when not moonlighting as a grief counselor, was a lactation consultant and told me that cabbage leaves, especially when kept in the freezer, would help relieve the throbbing of milk-engorged breasts. I first felt the familiar pressure and hot stinging in my chest while still in the hospital, my breasts filling up with milk for a baby who would never drink it. I nursed Alex for eleven months and couldn't wait to cuddle with this baby at my breast, too. Candy's advice, at first, sounded ridiculous, but I was willing to try anything to make this painful reminder go away as soon as possible.

Sitting on the couch wearing frozen cabbage leaves perfectly molded to my breasts, I looked like Wonder Woman gone vegetarian. My brother's girlfriend raised her eyebrows and laughed at me, and I laughed too, for the first time, it seemed, in a week.

Alex and her four-year-old cousin, Andrea, pushed the Little Tikes minivan around the cramped living room, Alex clinging to two pacifiers in her mouth—a habit we had let her fall into during the past week. "Do you know what Andrea said when I told her Auntie Monica's baby died?" asked my sister-in-law. I shook my head. "Well, she can just go to the store and get another one!" I smiled, wishing it was that simple.

Someone handed me a letter that had just arrived from the county coroner. "I wish to extend my deepest sympathy over the loss of your loved one, Miranda Novak. We recognize that this is a difficult time for you." The letter gave instructions on how to purchase extra copies of the certificate of fetal death. The problem was, I didn't need more pieces of paper telling me how she had died. I needed to know where she was now. I needed to know she was still with me.

11

On November 1st, All Saints Sunday—the day to remember those who have died during the past year—Al and I sit in church waiting for the service to begin. I hold my breath and quickly scan the alphabetical list of names inserted in the bulletin. Of course, I haven't forgotten her. I've been searching for Miranda ever since the shock of her death wore off. A friend had recently urged me to go with her to see a psychic. "It'll be fun," she promised. The promise of fun held no interest for me, but I had ulterior motives and agreed to go.

The woman lived in a small, ordinary suburban townhouse. Upstairs in a converted bedroom, the middle-aged woman with pouffy hair and glasses, wearing a flowing purple outfit, asked me to sit down across from a small desk. When she pulled out the Tarot cards, my defenses went up. It wasn't what I was expecting. She asked me to choose cards randomly—which went against my logical, methodical nature that never did anything randomly—and began telling me details about myself and my life.

"You're having an alignment problem," she said. My eyes widened.

"My car is pulling to the left. It needs an alignment," I confirmed.

A few Tarot cards later, she said, "You're concerned about a situation involving a fence."

I chuckled and explained we might be searching for a new house soon—since the Houston job still hadn't materialized—and were hoping it would have a fenced yard for Winston, my German-shorthaired pointer who's been boarding with my parents ever since I got married. She told me she didn't see a fence in my near future, which disappointed me. She then went on to describe the house we would buy: open floor plan, bay window, hardwood floor, planning desk in the kitchen, vaulted ceiling.

At the end of the hour, she asked if I had any questions. I was hoping she would be the one to bring up the real reason for my visit. I took a deep breath. "I recently lost a baby," I told her, my throat constricting as I forced the words out. "Is there anything you can tell me?"

She looked at me intently. "It was a boy?" she asked. My heart sank.

"No, it was a girl," I answered quietly.

"It feels like there was some kind of problem with her heart," she said.

Only that it stopped beating, I thought to myself. "I don't know, we didn't do an autopsy. I don't think so, though. It was a cord accident," I explained.

She had no concrete information, and I told her it was okay, I was just wondering. "Do you want to know if you'll have other children?" she asked. I nodded.

"I see a little boy, with light-colored hair."

I left with at least some hope for the future, but Miranda was nowhere to be found in this suburban townhouse of an ordinary psychic.

The church pianist plays softly in the background, and Al puts his arm around me while I scan the bulletin insert. Halfway down I see what I'm looking for. *Miranda Novak.* I breathe a sigh of relief and regret—glad she hasn't been accidentally omitted, but sorry that my baby is on this list. Most of these people lived long lives. Miranda and I have both been cheated—I as a mother, she as a human being.

When you lose a baby, you grab for whatever acknowledgement you can find, and reach far to fill the holes where the memories should have grown but never had a chance to take root. Today, we sit in a church to see our daughter's name in print and hear her name spoken.

"Miranda Novak," calls out the reader during the service, continuing on with dozens more names. I smile with a strange satisfaction and pride, as if Miranda has just graduated.

In the car, Alex shows me the cross she made in Sunday School with the words "Jesus Loves Me." The bulletin insert with Miranda's name in print is a pitiful keepsake in comparison, but a keepsake nonetheless, and I carefully lay it in Miranda's box when we get home.

~ ~ ~

One week later, my parents take care of Alex so Al and I can take a break from work, bills, and basal body temperatures. We fly to Clearwater, Florida, hoping to rekindle the fun and intimacy our marriage has lost since Miranda's death. Walks on the beach and quiet dinners work their magic–until I get my period and with it the frustration of knowing another month has gone by unfruitful. It's been almost five months since Miranda's death, and I had fully expected to be pregnant by now. Our sex life has lost all spontaneity; it's become a mission with one purpose. Last month's chart says we crammed two months worth of sex into one week. I don't know what more we can do. I go home disappointed and distraught, anxious for the next support group meeting.

~ ~ ~

"Did anyone see the news last night about the baby they found in a dumpster?" asks Beth at group. "That makes me sick!"

"What about the cocaine addict who delivered a baby in jail last month?" says Heidi.

"Those people don't deserve to have children. Their babies should be given to people who want them, who would love them like we would!" says Darlene.

"I don't watch the news anymore," I announce. "I can't even stand to see a parent yell at or spank a child in the store. And I used to be one of those parents."

The emotionally charged subject of child abuse and neglect is practically unbearable to everyone in the circle, and talk abruptly changes to the upcoming holidays.

Nobody in the room feels like they have anything to celebrate, and there's a general sense of dread connected with the thought of trying to keep up appearances for family's sake.

The most popular solution is to get out of town, preferably to somewhere tropical. I know two couples who have done just that. Jeff and Rachel escaped to Hawaii after their first pregnancy ended in miscarriage—it's where they conceived Sean. Another couple I know conceived their daughter in Hawaii after their infant son died. "Hawaii is a good choice," I say. We all laugh, but it's not a bad idea.

"Allow yourself to be selfish. Bow out of family celebrations if you aren't up to it," says Dawn.

"We were so excited about having our new baby with us and opening presents on Christmas morning," says a new mom. "We don't know what to do for her now."

"I hang stockings for the kids," Dawn says. "And they each have special ornaments we hang on the tree. We also go to the cemetery to decorate."

Someone suggests buying gifts for children in need with the money we would have spent on presents for our babies.

"We took gifts to the people at the hospital who took care of our babies," says Dawn. "The Maternity Unit got tins of popcorn. We wanted to do something different for the NICU (Neonatal Intensive Care Unit) that would benefit other babies and were told babies were responding to music, so we brought three cassette players, each with the name of one of the triplets on the back. Andy explained to the nurses why we were there, while I sobbed."

After an hour of small group talk following the meeting, Beth says, "Hurry up guys, let's go, Omega stops serving at 11:00, we won't get our French toast and beer!"

~ ~ ~

At Omega, our waiter walks up and turns out to be Tony from the last time we were here. He doesn't remember us until Beth places her order for French toast and beer. Tony's face lights up with recognition as he looks around the table, grins, and shakes his head.

After we place our orders, Beth tells us she has an idea for a new store in her town. "After Josh died, I was constantly looking for mementos to bring home, things I could give to people to remember him by, or things I could give to other people who were grieving. My store will have sympathy cards, birth and death announcements, artwork with serene scenes and comforting quotes or verses, angel statues, inspiring music for memorial services. I'm going to call it Good Grief. And I know the perfect location: downtown, right next to the funeral home."

"Well, what do you think of that?" asks Heidi, looking at the rest of us.

"Beth, that's perfect," I laugh.

"Maybe you can give me a job," says Dawn.

"I'll work there, too," says Darlene.

"But Darlene, there won't be any babies there for you to take care of," I tease.

"That's fine with me. I'm working thirteen-hour days at my nanny job. I could use a break."

"*Good Grief.* That would make a good name for our club," I tell everyone, laughing.

"Yeah, the club none of us asked to join," says Dawn.

"The club all of us would be seriously lost without," says Heidi.

~ ~ ~

As we make our way out to the parking lot, Dawn tells us about her conversation with a new mom after the meeting. "She said to me, 'I can't imagine what you must have gone through, losing triplets. I don't know how you handled that. My experience was nothing compared to yours!' And I told her, 'I was thinking the same thing about you.'"

12

When Dawn and Andy began dating in 1989, the twenty-eight-year-old already knew she had fibroids—common, noncancerous tumors in the uterus that were suspected to sometimes cause miscarriage by preventing implantation. The doctor was watching them for changes, and they were growing rapidly. "If you're going to have kids, you need to have them as quickly as possible because I don't know what's going to happen. We can do surgery down the road, but I don't know if you'll still be able to get pregnant," he told her.

"Can I at least get married first? It might help with the family," she said with a smirk.

"Yeah okay, I guess that would be alright," he laughed.

After the wedding and one year of trying to conceive with no results, she began a regimented routine of medication and artificial insemination. Despite all efforts, she still wasn't pregnant.

Their next hope was in-vitro fertilization (IVF), in which the egg and sperm are joined outside the mother's body and then transferred to her uterus. After one attempt, an ultrasound showed that three embryos had implanted; Dawn was carrying triplets. Her fibroids made her the least likely candidate for IVF to work, yet she was the only successful triplet pregnancy at the clinic that month. It was September of 1993; the babies were due the following June, the day after her 33rd birthday. With the support of Andy and her doctor, she went on medical leave from her job at the hospital where she worked as a labor and delivery nurse.

Eight weeks into the pregnancy, she began passing large blood clots in the bathroom. Panic-stricken, she was sure her pregnancy was over. Her obstetrician (OB) sent her to a high-risk facility for an ultrasound. They were full and wouldn't see her that day. Furious, she left and went to her infertility clinic. They performed the ultrasound for her and everything looked fine.

Dawn transferred to another group of obstetricians that specialized in high-risk pregnancies and every two weeks made the forty-mile drive for her appointment and ultrasound. At any hint of a problem or the sight of pink-tinged blood, she and Andy rushed to the doctor's office only to be told that everything was fine, go home and lie back down.

At a neighborhood party, Dawn learned that a woman on the next street over had triplets, and she called the mother to ask if she could come over and see what it was like to care for three babies. She came home excited to tell Andy everything she had learned. Soon after, Dawn began going to triplet meetings with her new friend.

At twenty weeks she was put on bed rest as a precaution. She was allowed to sit up and eat a meal for fifteen minutes at a time, and could go to the bathroom and take an occasional shower, but nothing else. The mother of the triplets called every Monday to see how she was doing.

Three weeks later, as Andy was getting ready to go to work, Dawn suddenly felt a gush of warm liquid between her legs. "Oh my God, Andy, my water bag just broke!" she yelled. Andy ran in.

"It's probably not your water bag, don't worry, I'm sure everything's okay."

"I know it is, I know it is! Call the doctor, call the doctor!" she cried in a panic.

"Yep, your bag is broken. It doesn't look like a good situation," her doctor confirmed. He put her in a wheelchair and pushed her over to the hospital obstetrics unit where she was met by a perinatologist.

"Twenty-three weeks is not a good time to deliver. If we can get another week out of you, you have a slightly better chance. If we can get three more weeks out of you, the chance of these babies surviving skyrockets. But we'll have to wait and see."

A young woman came in and introduced herself as Trish, the hospital chaplain. Dawn wasn't in the mood to be bothered with prayer; she just wanted to be left alone. Trish got the hint and left.

Dawn was afraid to move for fear of increasing contractions, but by six p.m. they were coming on strong and she grabbed the sheets in pain. She had dilated to four centimeters. "Get her on the cart and get her to L & D now!" the resident yelled to the nurses who rushed to get her to the Labor and Delivery unit. "Don't push, don't push!" the residents told her. She knew not to push, but it didn't matter; a baby was coming and there wasn't a thing anyone could do about it.

Medical staff came out of the woodwork. There were so many people around her, Andy was trapped in the corner of the room watching helplessly. After two pushes, a baby slid effortlessly from Dawn's body. They quickly held the baby girl up for Dawn to see and then rushed her to the Neonatal Intensive Care Unit (NICU).

"This doesn't usually work, but we're going to try to stop your contractions, put a stitch in you, and see if we can save the other two babies," said the doctor. They tilted the bed, leaving her head down at an angle and her buttocks and feet up high, legs spread apart.

"Please don't move me. I don't want to move," she said, oblivious to the burn mark that was forming on her skin from the heat lamp.

"We're going to start you on some medication," a nurse told Dawn.

"You mean stuff that's going to make me feel like shit."

The nurses looked at each other. "Are you a nurse?"

"Yeah."

"What kind?"

"Labor and delivery." Their eyes widened. Dawn knew what was going on; they were going to have to level with her.

They moved Dawn into a comfortable position and she began to feel better. The monitors indicated that the other two babies were doing fine. A nurse gave Andy a Polaroid of the baby to bring to Dawn. Someone had called their priest in, and he asked if he could say a prayer with them. "Fine," Dawn answered. As soon as he left the room, Dawn's second bag broke. *Well a lot of good you did me.* Now look what's happened!

Dawn hit her call button and once again they all came rushing into her room, setting up for another delivery. The second baby girl slid out, let out a small cry, and was rushed to join her sister in NICU. Suddenly, Dawn's third bag broke. The baby boy began to come out breach and his head was stuck inside the birth canal. Dawn was so panicked, she couldn't comprehend what they were telling her to do. Six minutes later, she managed to push the baby out. He had a knot in his cord, and one minute later their son was pronounced dead.

"We'll do everything possible for the girls, within reason. When it looks like what we're doing isn't making any progress, then we need to decide if it's really worth it. They have a chance, but it's not a very good chance," the doctor told them.

"What exactly are their chances?" asked Andy.

"One in five."

To this new father, that meant his daughters were going to survive.

~ ~ ~

Dawn and Andy kept their baby boy, named Christopher, in the room with them for almost an hour. Andy was back and forth between his wife and his daughters, whom they had named Katlyn and Amanda. She held her son and cried. "What are we going to do?"

As a labor and delivery nurse, she had experienced the awkward feelings watching a family after a pregnancy loss or infant death and saying to herself, *Oh God, just get me out of this room.* She remembered the day she was caring for a family that knew they were delivering a baby with a fatal birth defect. After the baby died they bathed and dressed him in a christening gown and took family pictures. "This is the strangest thing I have ever seen," Dawn had whispered to the doctor.

Now she was on the other side of the fence. Now she understood the importance of these first and last moments with a child. *Why, God, did I have to learn it this way?* As she held her baby boy for the last time, she looked down with sadness. There was nothing she could do for him now, but she still had two baby girls fighting for their lives on another floor.

~ ~ ~

The next day Trish, the chaplain, came back and stayed with them. Dawn's earlier resistance to Trish was quickly fading. "Maybe you could put in a few good words for us," Dawn said glancing up to the ceiling and then back at Trish.

"Well, sometimes He and I don't get along, so maybe I'd better not say too much. I don't want to make things worse." Trish's humor lightened the mood and made Dawn realize that it was okay to be angry with God.

Andy was up and down, bringing new Polaroids to Dawn of the baby girls she hadn't been down to see yet. They lay in their isolettes under a heat lamp, sometimes wrapped in plastic to keep their body heat in. Tubes in their mouths connected them to ventilators to help them breath. Wires and IVs covered their bodies. The babies each weighed just over 1 pound and measured almost the length of a 12-inch ruler.

Even as young as the babies were, Dawn and Andy were surprised at their children's family resemblances. Katlyn had Andy's nose and dark hair. Amanda was a good mix of both Dawn and Andy, but with very little hair. Christopher was the spitting image of Dawn's father.

The NICU called to say Amanda was unstable and Dawn and Andy rushed down. "You can touch them, but the slightest stimulation can cause their vital signs to go up or down because their skin is so transparent and sensitive," a nurse warned. After much hesitation, Dawn began to lightly stroke her baby girls. Unable to hold them, she felt helpless. She resisted the urge to connect with them for fear of getting even more attached than she already had during the past five months.

"Talk to them," the nurse encouraged. She didn't know what to say or do, but finally gathered the courage to speak softly to one of her babies. When Amanda heard her mother's voice, her vital signs shot up. "See? She knows who you are."

"Oh, you're ripping my heart out," Dawn said with a tearful smile.

The girls had size on their side. They were as big as some of the babies born at twenty-six or twenty-seven weeks. But she knew time was a more important factor in their lives and they just didn't have enough of it.

"It doesn't matter what physical handicaps they have, as long as they make it through this, we'll deal with whatever we have to," Dawn told Andy. But deep inside, she knew her whole world was falling apart. She was haunted by her doctor's words: *You're a perfect candidate for a multiple birth.*

~ ~ ~

Back in her room, Dawn asked to have her son brought to her again. The nurse carried him in a small wicker bassinet with a half hood over the top, blue ribbon woven through it. He was wrapped in a tiny crocheted blanket. She lifted him out of the basket. He fit in the crook of her arm, from her palm to her elbow. She looked down into his tiny face and cried. His eyes were still fused shut and covered with dark bruises. "What would you have been like?"

She saw images of the people she had taken care of whose babies had been born too early. She never connected with any of them; it was her job, she did what she needed to do and didn't get herself emotionally involved. It was an uncomfortable situation to deal with.

Now her own babies looked like theirs. Now she knew what it was like for those parents.

They took pictures of Christopher wearing a tiny white christening gown made by a hospital volunteer. Both grandmothers took turns with Christopher in the basket, passing him back and forth, but neither grandfather saw him. "I can't, I just can't see him that way," Dawn's dad told her.

Several more times that day the NICU called to say Amanda's condition was deteriorating and they would do what they could. Each time Dawn and Andy made it downstairs, she began to stabilize again. She fought hard, always pulling through on her own without much intervention, and both girls made it through the night.

~ ~ ~

The next day, the NICU staff prepared to take Katlyn for x-rays to look for a suspected brain hemorrhage. Suddenly the room was filled with commotion. "We need help, we need help over here!" nurses yelled. Dawn, Andy, and her parents were ushered into a room to wait. The wait seemed like forever to Dawn who was hysterical.

One of the doctors came in. "We've been working on her for forty-five minutes, she's not responding. What do you want us to do?" They weren't prepared to answer that question and were once again flooded with emotion. They held onto each other sobbing, knowing there was no hope.

"Just let her go."

"We'll bring her to you," the nurse said. Dawn's dad panicked. He didn't want to see her, but he couldn't walk out on his daughter. The nurse came in and gently laid the baby in her mother's arms. Her tiny heart was beating slowly as she struggled to take her last breaths. Dawn held her gently and watched her too-tiny, too-short life slip away.

"Find Trish, find Trish!" Dawn cried. The nurse came back in with a Polaroid camera. Dawn asked for Christopher back so she could hold them together. Andy wouldn't let them take pictures of the two together; he felt the triplets should all be together or kept separate. They spent an hour with their little girl knowing that, because Dawn was being discharged later that day, they may never get another chance to hold her.

Amanda was still hanging on, and they gathered themselves together and focused on their last living child. Dawn and Andy lived too far to go home, knowing that if something happened, they would never get back in time, so they stayed at the hospital as late as they possibly could. Trish made reservations for them at a nearby hotel, and it was close to midnight when they left the hospital and their baby.

~ ~ ~

The next morning, Dawn woke up with a feeling of relief. "We made it through the night without a phone call." Those words barely got out of her mouth when the phone rang.

"Amanda had another episode, but she stabilized and she's doing fine now. It might be a good idea if the two of you get over here as soon as you can, though" said the nurse. They rushed out, telling the front desk clerk they didn't know when they would be back. They were relieved to find Amanda doing fine when they arrived. When it was time for a shift change, they went up to the cafeteria to get some breakfast.

Dawn picked at her food. "I don't know what we're going to do Andy." They decided to go down to the chapel for some quiet time and prayer, but before they could leave the table, the hospital paging system came on, and they heard their names being called to the NICU. "Oh, no! We'll never get the elevator!" They were on the tenth floor and had to get quickly to the second floor, but there was always a long wait. They ran to the elevator, pushed the button, and it opened immediately, as if it was waiting for them.

When they arrived at the NICU, they prepared to scrub and put gowns on, a mandatory procedure to enter. "You don't have time, just get in here!" Doctors and nurses worked desperately to keep her alive. "We've been doing this for five minutes." Finally, all efforts were stopped and Andy and Dawn watched as they disconnected the baby from her lifelines, picked her up and gently placed her in her mother's arms. No words needed to be said; it was time to let Amanda join her brother and sister.

Dawn had delivered three babies and within three days watched helplessly as each of her children took their last breath on earth. The horror of it all was too much to comprehend. They called family and the church to say they had lost their last baby, but Dawn told her family to stay home. She just wanted to be left alone.

They came home from the hospital and went directly to a family birthday party. She didn't want to go, but everyone encouraged them to come and be with the family. Andy's sister had lost a baby to SIDS, so Dawn felt at least she would understand. She told herself she wasn't going to let anyone see her cry. But holding her pain inside hurt more than the pain itself, and she left there swearing she would never go to another child's birthday party on the anniversaries of her children's deaths.

When they finally came home that night, exhausted and dazed, the reality hit her. *My whole life was supposed to be different and now everything I was supposed to be doing isn't going to happen. I was supposed to quit my job to stay home and take care of these children. What am I going to do?*

~ ~ ~

Now began the difficult task of planning a funeral. When Christopher died, the questions raced through her mind. *What if we bury him and then two weeks later one of the girls dies and we have to do this all over again?* Then they lost Katlyn, and the two babies were kept at the hospital morgue waiting for their sister's outcome to be determined. Now Amanda was gone and Dawn knew there was only one way to do it. "They came together. They left together. They'll be buried together."

Andy didn't want a funeral at all, but Dawn persisted.

"Andy, let's have this funeral. Then we'll have everyone there and get it over with. Everyone can come up to us with their first reaction to us losing our kids and get those uneasy *What do I say to them?* situations over with at once," Dawn pleaded.

At the funeral home, they sat with one of the young funeral directors in the family-owned business. They were numb. He was uneasy. It felt like a business deal. "To be honest with you," he said, "I'm having a really hard time with this. I've never had to deal with this kind of situation before." *Like we have?*

Dawn ignored his comments. "It's very important that you have them in the right order in the casket. Christopher is self-explanatory. Katlyn has her dad's nose, and Amanda looks like both of us.

He looked at her like she was out of her mind. "Don't they have tags on them?" he asked.

"Okay, one of the girls has a clear dressing on her head. That's Amanda."

"That's all I need to know."

"Once you have them ready, I want to see them," she told him.

"Well, I'll tell you right now, we can't embalm these babies, because they're too premature. They're not going to look very good."

"I don't care. I still want to come in."

~ ~ ~

"I'm telling you, they don't look very good," warned the funeral director when they arrived for the wake.

"That's alright," she said and went in with her camera. The babies rested in a white casket cushioned by white satin pillows and ruffles, surrounded by dolls and teddy bears in colors of pink, yellow, and blue. Side by side, they lay in birth order, wearing crisp, clean christening gowns, extras that had been given to them by the hospital, allowing Dawn to keep the original gowns. Also placed in the casket were three photos: the house they would never come home to, the nursery they would never sleep in, and their parents who would never hold them again.

Emotions poured over her as her eyes came upon her children, back together again for the first time since leaving their mother's womb. Dawn never held all three babies at the same time; it was something she would always regret.

They spent a lot of time looking at the babies and taking pictures. The girls looked better than they had at the hospital, their skin more flesh-colored, less dark and bruised. The funeral director kept peeking in the room.

The casket was closed for the wake, but it was important to Dawn that everyone realize that three real babies lay inside, so above the casket stood a hospital certificate with their tiny footprints stamped in ink.

At the hospital, Dawn had shut out most of her family; trying to focus on the babies, she didn't want any distractions. Now she wished her sister and kids had seen the babies and better understood the scope of the tragedy.

Some of the family said it wasn't right to have a funeral and kept referring to the babies' deaths as miscarriages.

"Where are the babies? I want to see them. Where are they?" Dawn's four-year-old niece insisted. She had gotten so upset at the news of the babies' deaths that she tore her bedroom apart.

"They're in the box," Aunt Dawn explained.

"Well, why can't I see them?" she kept asking.

~ ~ ~

At the church, Dawn talked herself into the idea that she wasn't going to show any emotion, but during the ceremony, Andy's sister, whose baby had died, began sobbing. That triggered Dawn's sister to start sobbing, and finally Dawn lost what little control she had left.

The cemetery they had chosen for their children's resting place wasn't as scenic as the first one they looked at with rolling hills. But Andy's infant nephew was buried here, the plots were much more affordable, and it was closer to home. Unlike the other cemetery, this one had no restrictions about decorations. "You paid for that spot. Do what you want with it," the cemetery clerk had told her.

When Dawn arrived at the gravesite, it was covered in snow and ice from a recent snowstorm, almost forcing the cemetery to cancel the funeral.

The vault that would hold the casket had shiny gold plates with the children's names on them. "I wish I had my camera to take a picture of the gold plates," she kept saying, oblivious to the stares from everyone around her.

They went to a restaurant to have lunch with the family and ended the day at Dawn's house. "So what are we celebrating?" her confused grandmother asked.

~ ~ ~

Dawn was numb. She felt like damaged goods, blaming her faulty, fibroid body. *I've brought so much pain to Andy and the family. Why me? Why do I have all of the problems? What if I had gotten married younger? Did I wait too long to have kids?* She tormented herself.

The scene played over and over in her mind. It's the day before her water breaks. She's lying on the couch. She feels a sharp pain, but it goes away. She dismisses this pain, telling herself everything is alright.

If I had gone in at that moment would things be different? She would always wonder. "Don't do this to yourself," her doctor told her.

Walking away without a reason made it more difficult. What would happen if they tried again?

Upstairs waited a newly decorated nursery and three mattresses ready for cribs and sleeping babies. When Dawn and Andy returned the mattresses and cancelled the crib orders, they expected someone to ask why. Maybe the sales clerk knew not to ask. Surely this had happened many times before. But Dawn was disappointed because she wanted to tell everyone her babies were dead.

Invitations had recently been sent out for Dawn's baby shower and had started arriving in mailboxes when the babies were suddenly born. When Andy's family found out there would be no shower on that day, they scheduled a family birthday party instead.

One week later, Dawn's friend—the mother of the triplets—called. She had already called once, the day after Dawn came home from the hospital no longer pregnant and a mother only in theory, and listened with sympathy as Dawn told her what had happened. Today, Dawn shared her deep feelings of guilt over her body's failure towards her babies.

"I still feel guilty too," said her friend, "that I only got to thirty-three weeks and didn't get further with them."

But all of her babies lived and now she has three kids at home! How can she be saying something stupid like this to me? Dawn suddenly wished she could go away, far away, from the woman with triplets on the next block.

~ ~ ~

Ten days after burying the triplets, Andy's sister delivered her baby. Nine days later, another baby was born into the family. Dawn and Andy felt abandoned as the family busied themselves with the new arrivals. Dawn didn't want to see or hold them. She didn't want to know anything about them. "You're hurting their feelings by not paying attention to their babies," a relative told her. Against Dawn's wishes, she and Andy attended both baptisms. When Dawn was forced to buy baby gifts, she chose outfits she would never pick for her own children. In a sense, it was a form of therapy.

Emotionally, Dawn and Andy were at different ends of the world. He felt there was nothing more they could do. They had to move on. He was sad, but seldom broke down.

"For God's sake, can't you cry?" Dawn yelled.

"That's just not me."

"Well, then make it you!"

"I can't feel sorry for someone who feels sorry for herself."

"Andy, your life wouldn't have changed that much if the kids survived. You still would have gone to work every day, coming home at night to a house full of kids. My life was supposed to be the kids! I was going to quit work and be a full-time mother of multiples. My whole life was supposed to be different. Now I don't know what I'm supposed to do with myself!" she cried.

She was consumed with the babies. Every day before bed she said goodnight to her angels in heaven, sometimes waking suddenly in the night with, "Kids, I don't know if I said it, but I hope you have a good night."

She bought everything she saw in colors of pink, yellow, and blue. Anything with an angel and a baby, she bought that too. Andy just watched. Dawn was unconsciously compensating for her lack of memories by surrounding herself with what might have been. Her entire house became a shrine to her triplets: teddy bears with pink, yellow, and blue ribbons; angels in every room, always in groups of three; framed footprints and handprints; plates and poems hung on walls; vases and jars filled with dried funeral flowers lined the shelves. Photo albums overflowed with photos of the babies, the cemetery plot, and every flower arrangement sent.

But angel babies bothered her. *Don't people realize that an angel baby means that someone's child died?*

Dawn often spent time looking through her children's few belongings, which she kept in a large box in her bedroom closet. She saved every card: *Congratulations on your pregnancy! You're having a baby! With Deepest Sympathy… You're in Our Prayers…* She kept pictures her nieces and nephews had drawn.

But the most precious keepsakes were the ones that had been in contact with her babies' paper-thin skin. Christening gowns, blankets, hats, and a blood pressure cuff. Locks of hair from the girls' heads. She hadn't thought to ask for Christopher's hair; she couldn't remember if he even had much hair. She didn't get his handprints either; his fingers had already contracted and they couldn't open his fingers enough to print them.

Dawn was so obsessed with protecting her children's belongings that during tornado season she had Andy bring the box downstairs so she could grab it quickly and take it down into the basement with her if the sirens went off. One Tuesday, when she heard the alarms in the distance, Dawn grabbed the box and ran downstairs. A few minutes later, she realized it was only the monthly test siren that had gone off.

She ignored Andy's suggestions to get a cleaning service because she was afraid of an angel or keepsake getting broken. She laughed that she would have to follow the cleaning lady around the house telling her, "Don't touch this and don't touch that…"

A few reminders she kept with her at all times. One was a bracelet Andy had bought her for Christmas when she was pregnant. He had no idea what to get, so the sales lady helped him pick a stone. "Get her an amethyst because it's purple, for royalty, and your wife should be treated like a queen," she said smiling. An eerie feeling came over Dawn the moment she realized amethyst was the birthstone for February, the month the triplets had been born.

"Couldn't you have bought me an emerald or diamond? Then, maybe they would have made it until April or May," she told Andy, only half joking.

The night she lost her bracelet made by a friend with the kids' names on it, she rushed back to the restaurant they had just come from, asked the people sitting at her table to please get out of their seats, and crawled around on her hands and knees desperately searching. She was devastated that she never found it.

When she lost her special pin, the one with three tiny foot-prints on it, she searched until she found a jeweler who could get another one for her. She bought extra angel pins, too, in case she ever lost one. She wouldn't leave the house without her pins.

~ ~ ~

She was in a fog, trying to make it through each day. *I got through one day. Great. Can I make it through the next day?* She found herself crying at preschool graduations for her nieces and nephews, thinking *I'll never get to see this.* She was beginning to believe she would never be a mother. During the next four months, she and Andy didn't talk about another pregnancy. They knew there was a possibility she would never be able to have children if her fibroids had grown too severe.

She was jealous every time she heard her father-in-law tease other women about having another baby. She was surrounded by happy people. She didn't want them to lose babies, but she wanted everyone to know what it was like for her.

Like the cashier at the grocery store one day. "I'm pregnant now and I'm just so hungry!" she said. Visions of reaching over the counter and grabbing her by the throat ran through Dawn's mind. *Did I ask if you were pregnant? My babies are dead! Leave me alone!* But Dawn said nothing and quickly left the store.

Not only was she surrounded by happy people, but mothers with triplets were coming out of the woodwork. Her old church had them, her new church had them, her dad's cousin's daughter had them, a friend of her mom had them, and there was the set in her neighborhood.

Then one day, while sitting on the front porch, she spotted a large stroller coming down the street. The woman parked it in front of Dawn and introduced herself. "These are my triplets and she's eighteen months old," said the woman lifting her older daughter out of the stroller. "I just moved in across the street and blah blah blah blah blah—" The eighteen-month-old took off and the woman ran after her, leaving the triplets sitting in front of Dawn who was about to lose it. Dawn lived on a dead end street and there was only one way out: right past the triplets' house. She was furious.

"You should be happy those kids were born healthy. Would you rather see their names written in stone like ours?" Andy asked her.

"Well, no, but I also don't want to see them living across the street from me. That house isn't big enough for them, anyway."

"What do you want them to do, move?"

Yes! she wanted to yell.

Now there were two sets of triplets in her neighborhood and she was left out. Being pregnant with triplets was like a membership to an elite club, and suddenly her membership had been revoked without warning or cause.

~ ~ ~

At her six-week check-up, Dawn's doctor said his partner felt absolutely terrible. "He sees you one week, tells you everything is fine, and the next thing he's delivering your babies and you lose them. He just doesn't know what to say to you." The doctor had practically run out of the room after each delivery, putting his head down and silently passing Andy in the hallway.

"If I ever get pregnant again, all I can say is you better have the hotline ready for me, because I'm going to be on it every few minutes."

"Don't worry, you wouldn't be the first. By the way, your bill is covered. Don't worry about it." Hospital charges had exceeded $50,000, and her doctors wrote off everything the insurance didn't cover.

Dawn's six-week maternity leave was up, but she couldn't go back to Labor and Delivery. She still blamed herself for losing the triplets and was constantly tormented by the same thought: *I'm a nurse. Why didn't I know something was wrong?* She got a doctor's order putting her on light duty, and the hospital put her in an office to file papers. Walking past the hospital nursery, she stopped suddenly at the sight of the new wallpaper border decorating the large, bright room. It was the same border she and Andy had put up in the triplets' nursery. *Oh my God, they're following me,* she whispered.

~ ~ ~

The months rolled by, and that fall, Andy and Dawn attended a family wedding. The date had been chosen to allow all the pregnant women in the family, including Dawn, to have their babies before the wedding. Dawn was seated with the parents of a pregnant bridesmaid, whom everyone was making a big deal about. Dawn rolled her eyes.

How exciting, blah, blah, blah. Why not just feed me to the wolves, because it would be less painful. The bridesmaid's father was looking at the footprint and angel pins on Dawn's dress. "What are those pins you have on?"

"They're for my kids."

"Oh yeah, I heard about that. That was kind of sad."

The wedding party introductions began and everyone clapped and whistled. He looked at Dawn again. "How come you don't smile? What's the matter with you?" She got up and ran into the bathroom crying. Everyone looked at Andy, wondering what her problem was. He went after her.

"I can't do this! The kids were supposed to be here. I don't want to be here, let's just go!" she cried. But Andy was in the wedding party. They couldn't leave.

Dawn felt at odds with everyone, even Andy's sister who had lost a child. "You never say anything about my baby that died," she had said one day to Dawn. "And you don't ever bring your triplets up."

"I didn't even know you when your baby died," said Dawn. "And my babies lived such a short time, I have nothing to bring up. Sometimes I think you people don't even know their names or their birthdays."

"How can you say that?"

"Because that's how I feel!"

"Well, you should have come to us and told us you needed something."

"We were the ones hurting. Why do we have to reach out to everybody? You should be coming to us. When other family members die, everyone goes rushing over there with cookies and spends time with them and wants to talk with them. But everyone's avoiding us like we have some kind of disease they're going to catch."

"I'm sorry you feel that way. When I lost my baby, I sought out people and let them know how I was feeling."

"Well, that's you, not me," said Dawn. She felt like she was being accused of failing to follow proper protocol for death and grieving.

They had followed some of the family ethnic traditions and then were told it wasn't appropriate because these weren't real babies, they were miscarriages. Dawn was furious. Being a nurse, she knew the term "miscarriage" medically referred to babies who had died before twenty weeks gestation, most often in utero. Not only had her triplets been born at twenty-three weeks, two of them lived for several days. It seemed like the family had forgotten. Andy put it all behind him, but Dawn never could, and it would be almost two years before Dawn would pay any attention to the new babies in the family.

Dawn's parents, on the other hand, began telling people they had nine grandchildren, "six with us and three that aren't." She appreciated their intentions, but their efforts became overbearing. They made weekly trips to the cemetery and insisted on coming to Dawn's house every week, whether she wanted them there or not. They were constantly buying things in memory of the kids: pins, angels, ornaments, stuffed animals. She needed more space to herself; she needed to have some special things just for her and her babies.

~ ~ ~

Six months later, Dawn went back to her nursing job in Labor and Delivery, but only twice a month, just enough to keep her nursing skills up. *I have to try. I have to know whether I can do this or not. I liked my job before. I can't just quit without giving it a try.* But her self-confidence was gone. Every time a baby had even the slightest problem, she second-guessed herself, breaking into a panic-stricken sweat. *Please don't die on me,* she prayed.

Some of the other nurses sensed she was having trouble. "Tell us what you need. What will set you off, so we can step in for you?" they asked. But not everyone in her department was so sensitive.

"Why did you even have the doctors work on the babies at all? Why didn't you just let them go?" asked one of the older nurses who had been shoving patients Dawn's way to bring up her skills that had suffered during her absence.

"They were my kids. What was I supposed to do? You hang onto every last hope you have. If there's a one hundredth of one percent chance that they'll survive, you take it!"

Dawn worked at the same hospital with Pat Vaci, and Pat encouraged her to come to support group meetings. Dawn felt she didn't need that kind of help. She thought support groups were for basket cases. "I'm fine," she told herself and others. But she wasn't. She needed a place where she could talk about her kids. She finally gave in to Pat's encouragement and began coming to meetings.

A year went by and Dawn watched people come and go. *I don't understand. I'm a veteran and these newcomers are going off and having babies while I'm still sitting here waiting.* Dawn stayed connected to the support group because she didn't know if she would ever have other children, and it was her way of keeping the kids alive in her memory. But sometimes she felt hopeless, stuck in the emotions.

"You may not notice it, Dawn, but you've come much further than you realize," Pat told her. "You've grown a lot from this." Pat helped Dawn understand she could keep her memories alive without holding onto the emotions—she could start focusing on other things. Dawn wondered if she could focus on anything other than having another baby.

13

For the first time, the Ray Conniff Singers belting out their 1965 version of "Here We Come A-Caroling"—a record I've been listening to with my mom since I was a little girl—has failed to get me in the Christmas spirit.

This holiday season will have to settle for whatever I can give, and what little that is will revolve around Alex. How sad it must be, I realize, for my friends Dawn and Darlene, who have to endure the festivities without any living children, relying on the Christmas memorial service at the hospital as one of their holiday highlights—the memorial service I've decided to forgo, trying to focus on those I do have to share the holidays with instead of the one I don't have.

I haven't blocked Miranda out; I've simply chosen to keep her near to my heart in a quiet way, buying her a teddy bear stocking to hang on the mantel and replacing the blinking star tree topper with an angel.

I spend my days sitting by the Christmas tree wondering what Miranda would be like if she were here. She would be six months old. Probably sitting up by now, just in time to have presents put in her lap. Of course, she wouldn't know what to do with them, so big sister Alex would have to help with opening. And then we would be pulling bits of wrapping paper out of the baby's drooling mouth and hands.

I spend my nights writing out Christmas cards, finally telling long-distance friends about Miranda's death, since I couldn't pull myself together enough to send birth announcements in the summer like Beth and Heidi did. I haven't bought Hallmark this year; instead I've chosen a card designed by a bereaved mother. On the front is a black and white sketch of a little girl catching a snowflake on her mitten. On the inside I write, *In Peaceful Remembrance of Miranda Blair Novak, June 20, 1995.* After signing our names, I add an angel stamp in gold ink to represent Miranda, an idea I've borrowed from Heidi.

Cards flood back to us with notes and prayers of sympathy. I'm floored by one particular letter.

> *Dear Al, Monica, and Alex,*
> *I'm so sorry to hear of the loss of Miranda Blair. Please know that you and she are in my thought and prayers. I hope you can get through this Christmas and the days ahead, reflecting on your bounties and blessings instead of your loss. It's tough, I know, and words just fail me at this point. I wish I could express the sadness I feel for you, my close, good friends, in the face of this tragedy. You'll have good days and not so good ones, but eventually the good ones will prevail. No doubt you've already moved on to better things, save for the occasional quiet look back. I hate to bring it all back by sending you this note, but I couldn't let this pass without offering you my sympathy and support. Please hang in there and look forward to brighter days. I wish you strength, serenity, and inner peace. It's really true, time and friendship are the great healers. Bide your time, look forward and know I'm here for you.*
> *With love, John*

John is an old friend of Al's from his school and rock band days whom we haven't seen in years. I'm amazed at the depth of compassion and wisdom from a single man I've only met once, who has never had children of his own.

On Christmas Eve, the church altar is filled with bright red poinsettias, one of which we have purchased in memory of Miranda— one of the few things I can think to do for her. After the service, we come home with our poinsettia and bulletin insert with Miranda's name in print.

Christmas morning, when Alex is finished opening her presents, Al hands me a gift. I unwrap a small ivory and red book with a gold star etched on the cover. *The Christmas Box* by Richard Paul Evans. I know the story has something to do with the loss of a child; it's the most personal gift Al has ever given me.

My gift to Al was equally personal and special this holiday season. His poem "Why is Everyone So Sad?" was chosen by Share Pregnancy and Infant Loss, Inc. to be published in the November/ December issue of their national newsletter, *Sharing*, after I submitted it to them in the summer.

In the afternoon, at a family gathering, one of my cousins announces she's pregnant. Many times I've fantasized about announcing a new pregnancy on Christmas Day. As I hug my cousin, I resign myself to the fact that I won't be adding my name to that list—the list of seventeen currently pregnant women I know. I know there are seventeen because I counted. Then I made a list to keep track of the due dates. I don't know why I think this is a good idea; it makes me miserable every time I have to add another name that isn't mine. It seems every woman of childbearing age within a thirty-mile radius is about to bear a child—except me.

But, it's a new year full of new chances and I'm feeling hopeful—until the day I get my period and sink to the floor sobbing. "Damn it!" I scream, remembering from my chart the number of times we had intercourse last month. Six times. *How much longer can this go on?* Seven months have come and gone, and I'm beginning to panic, almost certain I've run out of eggs or Al has secretly been sitting in hot tubs when away on business and has boiled his sperm to death.

When I call Dr. Ross to voice my concern, he tells me that in the perfect environment, with two very fertile people, the chances of getting pregnant are only about 20-25% each month. Al and I have been very fortunate until now. He tells me couples aren't considered infertile until they've been unable to conceive after one year, and then he reminds me how much physical and emotional stress my body has been through. I realize my expectations are too high and I breathe a sigh of relief. "If you aren't pregnant by next month, call me and I'll have you come in. Maybe we can help you along with something."

~ ~ ~

It's the second Thursday of January, and I'm anxious to see my friends and ask them how they survived during the holidays. Walking into the quiet north pavilion, I find it ironic that our support group meetings are held here in the hospital's Mental Health Center solely as a matter of room availability, yet the people who walk into a meeting do so hoping to claim back some piece, however large or small, of the mental health they've lost along with their babies.

On the elevator ride down, I strike up a conversation with another mother I've only recently met. I tell her about a book my mom gave me for Christmas two years ago that I rediscovered tucked away on a shelf. As I reread *Embraced by the Light* by Betty Eadie, the gripping account of her near-death experience, I grabbed my highlighter, fervently marking passages that seemed to be speaking directly to me, words I had casually passed over before my life had been forever altered. Slowly, the idea formed in my head: *Maybe Miranda chose to come here. And maybe it was her choice to leave. And maybe the spiritual reasons are more than my human brain can understand right now.* This is a new concept I hadn't considered before. *Chose to come here?* I never believed God took her away from me. I found no comfort in the thought that her death was random, with no reason or meaning whatsoever. This is the only explanation that seems to make any sense. Although it doesn't lessen my pain, it's an idea I can believe in.

"I hated the book and didn't find that theory helpful at all," says the woman as the elevator door opens, and she walks out missing the sight of my jaw dropping.

I sit down next to Beth in our circle of chairs and she leans over to whisper to me. "Dawn just had a miscarriage."

"I didn't even know Dawn was pregnant!"

"It was early. I think she was about six weeks."

Beth is the glue that holds us together, both individually and as a group. She's the hub that disseminates information to each of us. Beth always knows what's going on in everyone's lives because she makes it a point to stay involved through phone calls and visits. She cares as much about each of our struggles and successes as her own. Compassionate and supportive, never critical, she's always there when one of us needs her, even if it's 1:00 in the morning.

Dawn walks in with Andy as the meeting starts, so none of us has a chance to talk to her before the meeting. We all expect her to add the miscarriage to her introduction, but she talks only about the triplets.

There's a new couple here tonight. The woman, tall and slender with brown shoulder-length hair, wearing jeans and a sweater, has her head down and holds a tissue to her face, unable to speak. Her husband takes the cue and talks for the both of them. "My name is Jim, and this is my wife, Tracy. In November, we lost our son, Paul, at full-term. He was stillborn. We don't know what the reason was; the autopsy was inconclusive." Tears stream down Tracy's face, and our hearts go out to her, knowing the pain that's tearing her up inside. I'm immediately drawn to Tracy because our circumstances are so similar. I make a mental note to catch her after the meeting before she leaves.

After introductions, the floor is opened up. There's a lot of talk about the holidays and how everyone managed to get through them. "Christmas sucked!" says Beth. "It was really hard without Josh. When I finally accepted I was going to have another baby, I envisioned

Christmas time with Madeline and her baby brother. They were going to be dressed in matching outfits for our family Christmas card picture. Then it was Christmas and no baby." She tells us about their trip to Phoenix to spend Christmas with Jeff's parents. She orchestrated a ceremony on Christmas Eve with printed programs and candles, and made them all sing "Silent Night." She didn't care what anyone thought; she did what she needed to do.

Heidi's mom let her have Christmas at her house, and before Heidi would let anyone eat, she made the whole family do the same candle and song service that Beth was doing in Arizona.

"All year I've been buying stuff for David, who's five, because shopping is how I cope. But Christmas for him was like a Toys R Us giveaway extravaganza!" laughs Heidi.

"I had this newborn baby doll I was going to give Alex when I brought Miranda home," I tell everyone. "I thought we'd have fun taking care of our babies together. I hid it high on a shelf in my closet when I was pregnant and forgot all about it. When it got cold, I pulled down my sweaters and found the box with the doll in it. I cried and then put it back on the shelf, hoping I would still have a chance to give it to Alex some day. But every time I thought of it, I was reminded of the baby that never came home with me, so Alex and I wrapped the doll in a receiving blanket and sent it to a toy drive for abused children. Hopefully some little girl had a happier Christmas because of that doll."

Jim joins in frequently. He's good-natured with an obvious sense of humor, and we quickly take to him. He tells us a story about a stuffed monkey Tracy had bought for the baby during her pregnancy. After Paul died, the monkey became a symbol for Paul. "Most people have stars or angels on top of their Christmas tree. We have a monkey. We even took it on vacation with us," he says grinning and we all laugh.

Tracy sits next to him quietly crying, taking it all in, going through a lot of tissue.

"I'm glad I went through labor with Paul because that was all I could do as a mother for him," says Tracy, surprising us. "But I never unwrapped his blanket to hold him skin to skin, or give him a bath. I never asked to have him back the next day before we left the hospital. I never got a lock of his hair. I regret that we didn't have a full funeral service in the church with more people to honor him and his life, to let people know it wasn't just an unfortunate mistake, that he was a child, our son," she says and breaks down crying.

"Tracy, it's not your fault," says Beth. "A lot of us weren't given guidance. Nobody asked me, 'Do you have any questions? What's your support system at home? Would you like to see the baby one more time? Do you need help planning a funeral?' I regret not seeing Josh again after the delivery. I regret not inviting family and friends to the cemetery because they didn't acknowledge our loss. We didn't think a full funeral was acceptable for a preterm baby, but later learned from talking to other people, it would have been okay."

Darlene shakes her head. "Three months after losing the twins, after coming here and hearing that so many of you got to hold your babies, dress them, and baptize them, I wrote a five-page letter to our hospital's president saying that they really needed to train their doctors and nurses on bereavement practices because this messed me up mentally and now I feel like a loon," says Darlene. "They wrote back saying, 'Thank you for your input, you will be hearing from us shortly,' but I never heard from them."

After the meeting, I walk over to Dawn—Beth, Heidi, and Darlene right behind me. "Beth told me about your miscarriage. I'm so sorry. What happened?"

Dawn tells us about her and Andy's unsuccessful attempt at in-vitro fertilization one year ago after losing the triplets the previous year. Andy had asked Dawn, "How many times are we going to do this? How many times do we have to hit our heads against the wall before we say enough is enough?" "Andy, the doctor is so hopeful. He really thinks this can work for us. I can't give up until I know," Dawn had pleaded.

Last month, in November, they went in for another IVF. They were hesitant to tell family they were doing IVF again because of their reactions after the triplets died: "See, you shouldn't have been messing around with infertility. It should have been left in God's hands."

Several days later, her blood work came back positive for pregnancy. They were guarded, but elated, telling the family right away so everyone would have time to invest emotion into it and offer more support.

Her blood work had been off from the beginning, though, and when the hormone levels failed to increase as expected, she was told to be "cautiously optimistic." A six-week ultrasound showed an amniotic sac with an embryo measuring only the size of a five-week-old, the heartbeat still not visible, and they told her she most likely would lose the pregnancy.

This is never going to work. Once again, my body has failed me, she told herself.

Soon after, she miscarried. It was just before Christmas. They told the family what had happened so everyone would understand why they were acting strangely. Dealing with their families during the holidays was already difficult. Now, with another loss, everyone was walking on eggshells.

"Please don't tell the kids," she told her family, "because I don't want them to think that every time Auntie Dawn has a baby, it dies." After the triplets died, Dawn's nieces played "funeral": their babies would die, and then they would have a funeral for them. *Oh God,* Dawn thought, *we've damaged everybody.* She was afraid the kids would start thinking that if they came to her house they would die, too.

Losing her second pregnancy early on was difficult, but the emotions and grief were short-lived. Because she had never seen a heartbeat and her condition was guarded all along, she didn't have as much invested into this pregnancy. It was never in her mind a definite thing, so she hadn't allowed herself to become emotionally attached to this new life. "That's why I didn't mention it in the meeting. I wanted all of you to know, but I didn't feel the need to share my feelings with everyone at group," she explains.

I watch for an opportunity to talk with Tracy and Jim. Beth and Heidi have the same idea, and when the couple is done talking with Pat, we all converge upon them like a flock of sea gulls. They remember that I also had a full-term stillbirth and we share more details of our stories. I'm concerned that they don't have a cause of death because, I share with them, I find some comfort in at least knowing why Miranda died. They surprise me by saying since there's no apparent genetic problem that might repeat itself in a future pregnancy, they're relieved not to have a reason.

We hug and tell them we hope they'll come back next month.

Dawn goes home with Andy, while Heidi, Beth, Darlene, and I head to Omega for a meeting of whom I now secretly refer to as "The Good Grief Club."

~ ~ ~

"Heidi has something to tell all of you," says Beth. Heidi grins.

"Are you pregnant?" I ask.

"Yep," Heidi says. Heidi's doctor told her to wait three months before trying to conceive. So July came and went, August came and went, September came and went. All summer, Heidi studied how to pinpoint ovulation, and by October, predictor kit in hand, she was determined to get it right. But conception didn't happen. What did happen was that Heidi cried every time she and Greg had intercourse, vividly remembering the feeling of Brittany's perfect little lifeless body sliding out of her.

"The next month I figured out I would ovulate while Greg was hunting in Wisconsin with a bunch of guys, so I said to him, 'Guess what, honey? I'm coming with.' I went hunting and not for wild game." Laughter erupts at the thought of Heidi sitting in a cabin, waiting to jump on Greg as he walks through the door with a deer slung over his shoulder. "So low and behold we got pregnant. Now I'm thrilled and sick as a dog."

Two hours later, it's time to go; the Omega is closing and we're getting kicked out. So we stand in the cold parking lot talking and laughing until our fingers go numb.

~ ~ ~

Once in my car, the quiet is filled with thoughts of Tracy. She spoke very little tonight, while her husband, Jim, shared and laughed. How clearly I remember those early days, yet it seems like a lifetime ago. *Hang in there, Tracy. It'll get better.*

As I pull out of the parking lot, I reach into my pocket for my gloves and find the wad of tissue I grabbed at the beginning of tonight's meeting; I know I'm getting better because it's still dry.

Yet, if only I were pregnant like Heidi...

14

By the end of 1994, Heidi's life had finally come together, or so she thought. She was newly married to Greg, newly pregnant, having conceived on their honeymoon, and Greg was going through proceedings to adopt her five-year-old son, David.

The following June, six months into her pregnancy, Heidi and her mom took David to Florida to visit Heidi's grandma and spend a day at Disney World—his last hurrah as an only child.

Driving back from dinner one night, Heidi and the baby played a game of keep away with the seatbelt: the baby kicked the belt, Heidi moved the belt, the baby kicked the belt, Heidi moved the belt again. As the next day went on, Heidi began to realize she hadn't felt the baby move, but didn't think much of it and drank a bottle of Mountain Dew remembering caffeine might help. Out for dinner that night, Heidi didn't feel good and started to worry. Her mom took her to the small hospital in Grandma's retirement community: *we'll hear the heartbeat and that will be that,* she thought.

The staff came in with an ancient-looking silver device, put some gel on Heidi, stuck it on and heard nothing. "This old thing," said the nurse. They weren't used to dealing with young pregnant women, and Heidi was now thinking they should have driven to a larger hospital in Tampa. "Well this probably isn't working right. We're going to send you for an ultrasound."

They wouldn't let her mom go in with her, they wouldn't let Heidi see the screen, and when the ultrasound was over, they wouldn't tell her anything because they had to call in the radiologist who was probably at home in bed.

Heidi and her mom sat in a curtained-off section of the Emergency Room (ER) and waited, and waited, and waited. Hours went by, nobody was coming to talk to her, the baby wasn't moving, and Heidi started to figure things out in her head just as the doctor pulled the curtain aside and said, "I'm sorry." She screamed and then broke down while her mom held her.

"Can't we give her something?" her mom asked.

"No, I don't want anything," Heidi insisted.

It was chaotic in the bright white room. None of the staff knew what to do. "She needs to get her doctor on the phone. Get her doctor on the phone!" ordered her mom. "She needs to call her husband. Get her husband on the phone!"

Her doctor in Illinois was kind and compassionate, said he was sorry and asked her to please call the office as soon as she got home.

It was in the early hours of the morning when she called Greg at home, waking him from a deep sleep, and told him that their baby was dead.

Heidi sat in her grandma's living room, staring at coverage of the hurricane that was hitting Florida and Christopher Reeve who had just fallen off his horse, while her mom made arrangements for her to fly home. She flew out alone before David even woke up; he was so excited about being a big brother and she didn't know what to tell him. On the plane she sat shriveled up in the corner, crying, oblivious to the passenger next to her.

At O'Hare Airport, Greg met her at the gate. She felt like she was in a movie scene: she gets off the plane; they walk up to each other, embrace, and everything else fades around them; only the two exist. At home, they crawled into bed together and cried.

That afternoon, her doctor shared with her that he and his wife, also an obstetrician, had lost a baby to stillbirth at twenty-nine weeks. He gave her the choice to go right to the hospital where another doctor was on call, but told her he would really like to deliver her if she could wait two more days.

She was glad she waited because it gave her more time to get her act together. She had never attended a funeral for a child and now had to plan one for her own; she didn't know what to do. When her cousin called and asked how she could help, Heidi told her to go to the library, get her some books, get her anything. There weren't any books to help her plan a funeral, but one of the books her cousin brought told her how important it would be to hold her baby. *Hold my baby? Alright.* She told Greg she would like his dad and dad's fiancée to be there. "Do you think they would like to hold the baby?" she asked.

He looked at her with surprise. "Hold the baby?"

Heidi and her mom went to the Beanstalk, a children's boutique in town, to buy an outfit for the baby to be buried in. The owner recognized Heidi who had shopped there a few times during the pregnancy. She told the owner her baby had died and she needed to pick two outfits, one for a boy and one for a girl, and asked if she could bring back the one she didn't use. It was the start of a special relationship between Heidi and the owner who knew something about her that other store clerks didn't.

~ ~ ~

"Have you been helped?" asked the ER receptionist who noticed Heidi sitting across from her.

"I'm waiting for Labor and Delivery to come down with a wheelchair," answered Heidi.

"Oh how exciting, you're here to have a baby!"

Heidi and Greg spent the night in the hospital, and the next morning after her parents arrived, her labor was induced. The next ten hours were a roller coaster ride for Heidi, one minute sobbing and the next minute laughing. Contractions were slamming her, one on top of the next, but when the doctor checked her at 6:00, she was only dilated to five.

Fifteen minutes later she was fully dilated and began screaming. The doctor ran back in and the baby slid out onto the bed. The doctor picked up the baby and walked out of the room. Heidi was relieved that it was over, but she knew a moment later that it was just beginning. "Was it a girl?" she asked when he came back in.

"You know, I didn't even look. They're washing the baby up. Give me a minute."

When they brought back the baby, a girl, she was wearing the white outfit with pink roses Heidi had bought and was wrapped in a blanket. She looked like a beautiful sleeping baby with red hair, red lips, and a little bruising. Heidi held Brittany while her pastor blessed her, and family came to say hello and goodbye.

All through the pregnancy she liked the name Brittany for a girl, but Greg was dead set against it because Brittany was the name of his best friend's dog. For the stillborn baby, Brittany was fine with him. "Whatever you want," he told her. The middle name, Rose, was chosen after a huge arrangement of pink roses arrived from Heidi's coworkers.

They took a lot of pictures, and after they brought the rocking chair Heidi had asked for, she rocked Brittany and sang to her, sobbing.

Her nurse answered all of Heidi's questions, cried with her, and later told Heidi she had lost two babies to miscarriage.

After they took Brittany away, David was brought to the hospital. She didn't know whether David should see Brittany and was encouraged by family to keep the five-year-old away from his sister— a decision she would always regret.

Although a teacher with early childhood background, Heidi didn't know what she was going to say to her son. He came in and crawled up on the bed, and the words seemed to come from nowhere, flowing out of Heidi's mouth quicker than she could process them. She explained the baby was born too soon. She was too sick and had died.

David sat quietly. "Does this mean I'm not a big brother?" he asked.

"Of course not. You'll always be a big brother to Brittany. And now you have a guardian angel."

Once home, Heidi's mom took her upstairs where she had twenty of her own outfits waiting for Heidi to try on; Heidi had no maternity funeral dress hanging in her closet and couldn't fit into anything else. She tried on outfit after ugly outfit. They weren't really so bad, but Heidi didn't want to find an outfit to wear to her baby's funeral, told her mom to pick one—*she really didn't care*—and went back downstairs, sat on a chair in her kitchen, and sobbed while her husband, parents, and in-laws cleaned the house to prepare for guests.

Greg and Heidi's dad went to the funeral home that night with things to put in the casket: pictures from their wedding, pictures that David drew, a toy that he bought for his sister, and a bible from a cousin. Heidi didn't go and later regretted her decision because it would be a closed-casket funeral, and other than a photograph, she would never see her baby's face again.

The day of the funeral, Heidi's milk came in; now she felt like a fat, bleeding, dripping mother who had to go bury her daughter.

At the funeral home, people came and said they were sorry, and there in the front of the room was a tiny, white casket that looked too much like a Styrofoam cooler with a baby inside, and Heidi could not believe this was really happening.

She sat on the couch, rows of people behind her, while the pastor said some prayers and other things she didn't remember. Then Greg's brother, who would have been Brittany's godfather, carried the baby down the steps, and Heidi suddenly had a vision of him tripping down the stairs and spilling the cooler.

They drove to the cemetery in a long procession like it was a dignitary's funeral. Heidi stood on the plastic green carpet while flowers and flowers and more flowers—the florist was a dear family friend—were unloaded and brought to the gravesite.

Brittany was being buried in the empty grave that belonged to Heidi's grandmother, and someday the baby would be removed and placed back in the grave on top of her great grandmother.

Heidi sat, once again, in the front row while the pastor said some words, people walked by, went back to their cars, and that was the end of it. Heidi walked up to the casket, fell to her knees, and sobbed.

Greg stood in the back dazed, holding David's hand. The adoption had just become final; Greg had gained a son and lost a daughter in the same week.

"Heidi, we need to go," her mother said, gently pulling her away.

Back at Heidi's house, people laughed and ate food from the grocery store party trays, and Heidi's journey of grieving and healing began.

~ ~ ~

Like any other new mom, Heidi took six weeks off from her job at the daycare center where she taught private kindergarten. Greg went to work, and Heidi and David drove to her mom's in a nearby town every day. They watched TV and ate bagels. Some nights she didn't bother to go home.

She didn't do anything but sit thinking about the baby girl who had no knot in her cord, no marks around her neck, and an autopsy that found no reason for the death; the baby was perfect in every way down to her miniature ovaries. They drew vile after vile of blood from Heidi to check for anything they could think of, but everything was normal.

Heidi coped by shopping. She bought new furniture. She bought pretty much everything she wanted. It became her mission to find red-headed angels, and she bought those too.

A family friend of her parents told Heidi about a support group that truly helped after her son was stillborn. Heidi called Beth, a friend she knew casually, who had lost her baby two weeks after Heidi. Heidi talked Beth into going, and Beth went under the impression that she was there to support Heidi, but Beth came to realize she needed the support just as much. The first few meetings were intense, but Heidi had Beth, and Beth had Heidi.

Over the past few months, Heidi and Beth had become close friends, practically inseparable, and spent hours on the phone every day or at each other's houses. Heidi, now pregnant again, was dealing with the mixed emotions of grieving Brittany, excitement for the new baby on its way, and the fear of losing this child, too.

15

February in Chicago keeps us indoors most of the time, and I realize I'm able to stay home now; the crippling fear of being alone has subsided. I've survived the worst months, despite not being pregnant. Although I think of Miranda often, the moments seem to be fewer and farther between. My focus now is on finding a new home. When the Houston job didn't come through at the end of 1995, Al told them to forget it and took a new job in Chicago. We put our townhouse back on the market and started looking for a house: a bigger one with more bedrooms for a growing family. Except the family isn't growing because I just got my period again. I'm too busy and distracted now to call Dr. Ross. Lynne, my friend at work, tells me she heard that drinking expectorant thins the cervical mucus and increases chances of conception. On the way home, I pick up a bottle of Robitussin.

For the moment, my arms aren't feeling so empty anyway. In December, my best friend, Kathy, delivered twin girls a month early, and they've finally come home from the hospital. Kathy and I have been like sisters since the sixth grade. She's the kind of friend you share all your firsts with: first sleepover, first cigarette, first cruise with your new driver's license. And the first friend you tell everything to: when you get your period; when you sneak behind the school to kiss a boy; when you've set a wedding date.

Last spring, right after I told her I was moving to Texas—which was harder than telling my mother—she told me she was pregnant with twins. She spent the next eight months so overcome with morning sickness that she could barely keep food down.

After Miranda died, I often found myself driving forty-five minutes to Kathy's house in Indiana. She was my safe harbor. I knew I could say anything, feel anything, act anyway I needed to. She cried with me, talked to me, asked questions, offered advice, and reminded me I was still alive, I was still a mother to Alex and Miranda, and she still loved me. And, she was one of the few pregnant woman I could be around who didn't drum up intense feelings of jealousy.

Now, I drive down to Indiana once a week to help her change diapers and give baths, giving her a break so she can take a shower or go to the store. I've accepted that this is the closest I get to having my own newborn right now.

I've relaxed somewhat about getting pregnant thanks in part to a woman I've met through the mail. She had posted a notice in *Sharing*, the national newsletter of Share Pregnancy and Infant Loss Support, looking for anyone who had a living child, had then suffered a stillbirth due to a cord accident, and was attempting a subsequent pregnancy. Her notice seemed to be speaking directly to me and I fired off a letter telling her our story.

She has a six-year-old daughter and has lost five babies: four miscarriages and one stillbirth. She's determined to continue trying until she has another baby in her arms. My letter had confided to her about my growing anxiety that my children, if I was blessed with another one, wouldn't be the age span I had always planned—two years apart. The "Marsha Brady" in me believed the closer in age my children were, the closer the sibling relationship would be, and month by month, I saw that gap widening. In my mind, my worries hardly compare to hers, but she's supportive and her words show no sign of judgment or comparison.

"Don't worry about the spacing," she says. "My sister and I are eighteen months apart and we have never been close. On the other hand, my two brothers, both more than a decade younger than me, are so much a part of my life, they're like my own children."

Through our correspondence, she's been reassured she's not alone in her struggle; I've realized my plans of child spacing hold no meaning or guarantees in the scheme of life, and I find myself letting go of another piece of the control I once thought I had.

~ ~ ~

At support group meetings, I begin to notice the faces of people who've been attending as long as I have are beginning to disappear and are being replaced with new faces. "Where are Janet and Scott?" I ask Pat.

"They're expecting again," she whispers. It's often the same story, just a different due date. Yet, I've been coming long enough to know some parents are ready to move on sooner than others regardless of whether there's a new pregnancy or not, and, in my mind, if you've healed enough to move on, that's a good thing.

Dawn's not here tonight, although I know she's not expecting. I'm glad to see Tracy and Jim back this month. Tonight is memory night. We've brought in photos and mementos of our babies to share with everyone. My regret and embarrassment grow as each person around the circle pulls out her treasures. They've put so much time and care into their babies' belongings; Beth and Heidi each have an entire scrapbook album.

When it's my turn, I pull out a photo from an envelope and feel compelled to make excuses. "I brought a picture taken of Miranda in the hospital. I see all of your beautiful things and feel guilty I haven't done anything more for Miranda. I guess it's because her things are all I have of her. Whatever I do with them has to be perfect. I'm afraid to make any mistakes, so they sit in a box on a shelf in my closet until I can gather the courage and creativity to do something special."

"Monica," says Beth, "don't be so hard on yourself. When the time comes, you'll know what to do."

"It's from the heart, and that's all that matters," says Heidi. Everyone nods, and I smile at them with gratitude.

"I'm glad the pictures captured the intense grief, because I don't feel that way anymore," says Beth. "At the time, I thought I would never be happy again. After I began to find happiness, then I felt guilty, as if I were betraying my son. But now I look at the photos, remember the pain and the grieving I did, and remind myself that I grieved enough."

Tracy sits quietly, watching us, occasionally fighting back tears. "You hope for the day when you can think of other things, when you don't think of your dead baby 150 times a day," she says out loud. She's putting too much pressure on herself to get on with life like it used to be. She expected to get back to normal and it isn't happening. That's one thing we've all painfully learned about life after the death of a baby; we never go back to normal. We're forever changed, and somehow we fall into a new normal.

Tracy continues. "Just being here, knowing that some of you were in the same place I am, seeing you coming around, not so sad, being able to find the good things about the experience of pregnancy and loss, to see that eventually there will be peace—it gives me hope."

At the end of the meeting, Pat tells us about the quilt project, explaining there are already three quilts hanging near the hospital chapel, each square handmade by a family who has previously lost one or more babies—Dawn's triplets take up two squares. Each square is as unique as each child would have been had they lived long enough for their personalities to shine through. She hands out blank quilt squares to each of us to take home and finish; our squares will then be sewn together by some gracious soul, and the quilt will be hung on the wall outside the chapel next to the other baby quilts.

~ ~ ~

"I just quit my nanny job," says Darlene, as we settle around a table at Omega for another gathering of "the club."

"I thought you loved that job," says Heidi.

"I did, but I started to hate the parents. They worked from seven in the morning until eight or nine o'clock at night. They were never home with their kids. So, I got a new job at a daycare center."

"She still needs to be around other people's kids," laughs Beth.

"Look who's talking. You've been babysitting somebody else's twin babies!" I tease Beth.

"Not anymore. I quit."

"Why? What happened?" I ask.

Beth tells us that after Christmas she told Jeff she was ready to try again to have another baby. Up until this point, she had been so heartbroken, she couldn't stand the thought of losing another baby and the doctor's diagnosis was uncertain: "Well, we really don't know. You might have incompetent cervix, but we're not sure because your first baby was full-term. You probably don't, but we can't really say. Maybe it was just a bad pregnancy." Incompetent cervix was a name doctors used to refer to the early unexplained opening of the cervix, frequently causing premature delivery.

"One month later, a pregnancy test came up positive," she says, but before we have time to get excited, she tells us she began bleeding a few days later. The bleeding lasted a week; the doctor called it a chemical pregnancy and said she was probably miscarrying. "I said to myself, *That's it, I'm done! No more kids! I can't take this anymore!*" she tells us.

"I couldn't handle the stress of everything, so I quit my babysitting job. But then I felt guilty about leaving the parents high and dry. I've been a mess ever since."

"Oh no, Beth, I'm so sorry," I tell her.

"It's okay. Maybe I should just count my blessings that I have Madeline and consider my family complete. Who needs the morning sickness, anyway? Just look at Heidi," Beth laughs.

16

During Beth's first pregnancy in 1993, the doctor told her not to be concerned about the spotting, and books she read said the contractions were normal. So Beth, a naïve first-time mother, accepted what she was told and delivered a healthy baby girl, Madeline.

Beth did the best she could to care for the baby while working part-time as a legal secretary, but Madeline, now sixteen months old, was wearing her down. Jeff had convinced her to move into a new house, a house that was above their means of income, a house that Beth didn't want in the first place. Their marriage was on the rocks, and somehow in the midst of it all, Beth got pregnant with Joshua. She wasn't happy about the unplanned pregnancy and sixteen weeks of morning sickness added to her stress. She considered quitting her job after the baby came, but how could she afford to stay home now with a big mortgage? Her anger with Jeff grew.

She spotted and cramped on and off from the beginning, but everything appeared fine. At sixteen weeks her morning sickness subsided, and soon after, she began to feel the baby move inside her. She finally began to feel happy about the pregnancy.

From twenty weeks on, she was going to the doctor's office almost every week because of spotting and contractions, and the doctor told her to take it easy. She found out she was carrying a boy.

At twenty-three weeks, she went in again, but this time, the doctor noticed that her cervix was softer. "I think I could push my finger through if I wanted to. You need to stop working and go on bed rest." Jeff took her downtown the next day so she could clean out her desk, but her boss was so anxious about her suddenly leaving, he had her work all day to finish things up before she left. She worked long and hard. That night she had more spotting. The next morning, she went back to the doctor with Jeff, who was getting ready to go out of town on business and didn't want to leave if there was something wrong. "You feel the same as you did a couple of days ago," he told her. "Just go home and lie down. I'm sure you'll probably go to term."

She went home and Jeff left town. Beth's in-laws, visiting from Arizona, were helping out with Madeline. Beth was on the phone telling a friend about her bed rest when she suddenly felt a gush of liquid between her legs. "Oh my gosh, I think I just peed my pants," she said and her friend laughed. She went into the bathroom, sat on the toilet and smelled her underwear trying to detect the smell of urine. She went back downstairs, sat down and more liquid leaked out. "Oh my God, I think my bag just broke."

"You need to get on the couch and call your doctor!" said her mother-in-law. Beth's hand shook as she dialed. "I think my bag broke," she told the doctor. There was silence on the other end. "I'm so sorry. I am so sorry," he told her. Beth began sobbing. "What do you mean, you're so sorry?" It felt as if someone had handed her a death sentence. "I'll meet you at the hospital," he said gently.

The contractions set in before she could leave the house. Her friends came over to watch Madeline, and her in-laws took her to the hospital. Stuffed in the back of their pick-up truck cab, she clutched the seat trying to lessen the bumps while they drove what seemed like eighty-five miles an hour. The doctor confirmed that she was leaking amniotic fluid. "We can't handle a twenty-three-week-old here. We're going to have to transfer you to another hospital where they have a high-risk nursery." You can get dressed if you want, and your in-laws can take you.

"My clothes are all wet from the fluid that leaked out while I was riding in the truck."

"I can order you an ambulance, if that's what you would rather have."

She called her sister-in-law, Joan, who had worked as a nurse at the other hospital and knew all of the doctors and medical staff. "I'm going to call ahead to the people I know. They'll be waiting for you," Joan assured her. "Do you want me to meet you there?"

"Thanks Joan," said Beth, "I would really like that."

The two ambulance drivers walked in. *Oh no.* One of the young men was a checker at the local grocery store. "What are you doing here?" she asked. It was awkward for both of them. Now Beth felt she had to keep up a good front; she couldn't cry or be scared or upset. Her natural reaction was to make people laugh, and they joked with each other during the drive as her in-laws followed in their truck. At a stoplight, Beth sat up and waved to them through the back window. She was in denial.

When the paramedics wheeled her out, she was met by a team of doctors and nurses, with Joan waiting in the background. Suddenly hit with the reality of her situation, she was overcome by fear. They rushed her into a high-risk Labor and Delivery room and hooked her up to the ultrasound.

"Okay, let's check this out," the doctor said. "Oh, there's a lot of fluid here, I don't think your bag broke." By this time, Beth knew her bag had broken, but the doctor sounded so positive. "This looks good. We're going to keep you overnight and check your fluid again in the morning." He did the same test the other hospital had done. It was positive. "Well, it is amniotic fluid, but it might just be a small little hole that could repair itself."

Beth was growing more upset. She and Joan had both tried to reach Jeff who was on his way to California. The airline paged him just as he was getting off the plane. When she told him what had happened, he panicked, asking one question after another. "Jeff, I don't know anything," she kept telling him. "We'll have to wait until morning." The next flight wasn't until 5:00 a.m. the next morning, and he found a hotel room so he could be by a telephone.

IV (intravenous) medication had stopped the contractions, but Beth lay awake all night in a room on the maternity floor feeling trickles of leaking amniotic fluid, holding her shrinking stomach, while the baby's movements changed from flowing to fitful.

Jeff arrived the next morning and they sat waiting. She had the sense to ask for ultrasound pictures, but with the large loss of fluid, it was difficult to distinguish the baby's body parts. He was still moving and kicking. He was still alive.

"One of three things is going to happen," the doctor told them. "You'll stay pregnant and carry the baby as long as you can, and we'll deliver you." She sensed that this was a slim possibility. "Or you'll go into labor. Or you'll start to show signs of uterine infection, in which case we'll have to induce labor and evacuate the uterus." He wouldn't give her any statistics. She sat quietly, trying to absorb what she had just been told.

Maybe she would be one of the lucky ones who continues through the pregnancy and delivers the baby successfully. But even if she remained pregnant, the damage to the baby from living without the amniotic fluid would probably be severe. "How long is it going to take, when will I know?" she kept asking. Not knowing was killing her. *If I'm going to lose this pregnancy, let's just lose it,* she thought. It sounded cold, even to her.

She got better answers from the nurses. "In your experience, how long has it taken someone to go into labor or develop an infection?" she asked each one who came into her room.

"The further you are from your due date, the longer it takes to go into labor."

"Well, is that three days or four days?" she pressed. One nurse told her to expect three days.

Beth sat in her bed, Jeff and his sister Joan keeping her company. When her lunch tray was brought in and put in front of her, she looked down at it as she felt the baby kicking. *I don't want this food, I don't want anything, what am I doing here?* It was a moment of clarity: life was dying inside of her and she sat trapped, waiting for it to end, watching everyone go on around her as usual. She broke down and sobbed uncontrollably and somehow managed to endure the rest of that day, miserably.

Saturday morning, she could still feel the baby's movements. Maybe things will go okay. She called her friends and family. "I'll probably be in the hospital all summer on bed rest," she told one after another. Her sense of humor peeked out once again as she joked with a friend. "Oh, this baby has been trouble from the very beginning. Just wait, he's going to be grounded as soon as he's born!" she laughed.

That night, one of her nurses walked in with a calendar. "I heard you tell someone on the phone you wished you had a calendar so you could mark off the days." Beth drew a sad face on the day her water broke and wrote her gestation on each box. Every day made a difference in this situation, and they talked in terms of gestational days instead of weeks: twenty-three weeks and three days, twenty-three weeks and four days...

The family settled into a daily routine: Beth did cross-stitch to pass the time, and Jeff brought Madeline after her nap. Beth grinned at her little girl when she walked in every day wearing summer outfits in sherbet colors of green, pink, and orange, her hair in crooked pigtails, climbing up into the bed with Beth so her mommy could read to her. Madeline didn't really understand about the baby, but sensed she had to be gentle. It was a special time, and Beth would sometimes cry when Madeline came to visit because she missed her little girl so much.

On Sunday, Father's Day, Beth prayed, "Dear God, please don't let him be born on Father's Day."

Early Monday morning, around 2:00 a.m., Beth was awakened by a strong contraction. She tried to remain calm. *It was just one contraction.* Twenty minutes later another contraction hit her, then another one twenty minutes after that. Beth called the nurse who wasn't too concerned about three contractions in one hour. At 5:30, Beth called Jeff. He was sleeping in an extra bedroom because he still hadn't made up his bed since his parent's departure. There was no phone in the extra bedroom, and sound asleep after being at the hospital late the night before, he didn't hear Beth's repeated calls.

"I hear you're having contractions," said the resident. "We're going to do a sterile exam," she said, raising Beth's bottom up onto a bedpan, spreading Beth's legs and using only a flashlight. It seemed archaic to Beth, but they had to be careful not to introduce bacteria. "You're dilated and I smell a foul odor which indicates infection. I'm going to send you over to Labor and Delivery." Beth broke down.

She frantically called Jeff again, screaming into the answering machine for him to pick up the phone. Finally, he answered. "I'm having the baby!" she screamed at him. "You need to get here!"

Leaving Madeline at home with a neighbor, Jeff arrived just as a neonatologist came in to talk to them. He told them that if the baby were at twenty-five weeks, his chances of survival would be 50-50. But at only twenty-four weeks, the chances were less. "As soon as he's born, we'll give him a shot of epinephrine. If his heart rate speeds up, that will be a good indication his heart is developed pretty well, and his other organs should be about the same. But if his heart rate doesn't speed up, what would you like us to do? Would you like us to use extraordinary measures to try and save the baby?"

The medical staff hadn't prepared them for this situation, maybe because they didn't want her to give up hope. But now she had to give the doctor an answer about extraordinary measures. *What extraordinary measures? An IV? Tubes all over his body? And then what would his chances be of ever being healthy?* Beth was totally unprepared and overwhelmed. "If you decide you want us to try to save him, he'll immediately be rushed out of the room and taken to the NICU where we'll begin working on him right away. But, he could die down there, and you wouldn't be able to hold him," he told her.

Beth was being forced to determine the fate of her unborn son in the midst of labor, a labor as painful as with her first child. She had been advised against pain medication to give her baby the best possible chance, and now she couldn't focus on anything. She and Jeff didn't want him to suffer from painful treatment. They agreed with the doctor that if initial efforts didn't prove fruitful, the medical team would back off and allow Beth and Jeff to give the baby what he called "comfort care," holding and loving the baby while he quietly died in their arms.

The mood in the room was somber. Beth silently focused on the clock. Jeff sat next to her, but she didn't want to be touched so he left her alone. The neonatologist sat on a chair with his head down, waiting. The nurses weren't cheering her on as they had during Madeline's labor and delivery. Beth felt the baby slide out of her body. "It's a boy," said the doctor, quickly clamping the cord and handing him off to the neonatologist. Beth began to sob, and when she looked at up at her doctor, she could see that he was crying, too.

Joshua had a tube down his throat and was bagged for ventilation, and she heard the "1-2-3, 1-2-3," counting of CPR. They worked on him for five minutes as she lay helplessly on the delivery bed with her legs up in stirrups, unable to see through her tears. "The baby didn't respond to the epinephrine. Do you want to hold him?"

"Of course I want to hold him," Beth cried, unprepared for the sight of her half-term baby.

As a woman walked in and introduced herself as the hospital chaplain, the doctor wrapped Joshua in a blanket and gently laid him on Beth's belly. She was shocked at first sight of him and a pang of guilt tore through her. He was gray, not the familiar pink, and his eyes were still fused shut. Jeff was a mess, unable to look at his son.

"Oh my God, he's so warm," she said. Weighing 1 pound 6 ounces, he was so small he fit in the palms of her two hands. His head, the size of a pear, had a light dusting of dark hair like his big sister had been born with. "He looks just like Madeline did, only smaller—the nose, the chin," she said to Jeff.

The baby didn't move, didn't cry. Every thirty seconds his mouth opened to take a breath. "Do you think he's in pain?" Beth asked a nurse.

"No, no he's not."

"Is he still alive?" Beth had to ask of her lifeless-looking son. The nurse came over and checked for a heartbeat.

"Yes, he's still alive."

Every time she saw his tiny lips open for air, Beth wondered if it would be his last breath. The doctors and nurses quietly left the room, leaving Jeff and Beth alone for the last few moments they would ever have with Joshua.

She passed him to Jeff who gently cradled Joshua in his hands, sat on a stool, and rocked him back and forth, looking down at his son. It seemed natural, as if this baby would be coming home with Mommy and Daddy soon, and for a moment she forgot her son was going to die.

A nurse came back two hours later and checked his heartbeat. She looked up at Beth. "I'm sorry, he's gone." Beth hadn't been aware of Joshua's final moment: his last heartbeat, his last breath.

"Oh, no," Beth cried, "I didn't tell him that I loved him!"

"Would you like to bathe him?" asked the nurse. Beth nodded. He had been delivered breech with his ankles crossed and his knees drawn up, and his body was covered with bruises. She gasped at the sight of him. His arms and legs were thin and unproportional to his head, his torso thicker than his bottom. "I don't think I can do this," said Beth, feeling another wave of guilt. The nurse took him out, and Jeff and Beth cried with the chaplain.

The nurse brought him back dressed in a white gown and wrapped in a special blanket. Beth wished she had her camera. Beth's pastor came in, and the chaplain took Polaroid pictures while the pastor blessed Beth and the baby.

Beth was ready to let him go. She had been crying for four hours and was exhausted. She didn't know what else to do. She didn't think to call family or friends to ask if they wanted to come and hold him. She felt so unprepared for this.

~ ~ ~

Friends and family came by that evening. Beth's mom had also lost a baby at five months term and had never been able to deal with it, so she didn't know how to deal with Beth's loss either. "Here, I brought you a Frosty," she said to Beth as she walked into the room.

"I don't want a Frosty. Do you want to see the pictures of your grandson?" Her mother glanced down at them, almost with a look of horror upon her face, and said nothing for the remainder of the evening.

The next day Beth was packed, showered, and sitting on her bed fully dressed waiting for three hours to go home. The shower was horrible, being in there with an empty belly and nothing to show for it. It was the first time she had felt with her hands the place where Josh had lived and grown for the past five months. Running her soapy wet hands over her flat stomach, she sobbed, missing him. For weeks afterwards, she broke down every time she showered, knowing that she should have been getting bigger.

"If you're in pain, take your Vicodin. Finish your prenatal vitamins. If you have a fever, call your doctor," said the nurse who discharged Beth, who also happened to be pregnant. Beth was given a pamphlet about grieving, a booklet for siblings called *No New Baby*, and a flyer about a support group.

"I think we'll have a private burial," Beth had mentioned to the chaplain earlier.

"That sounds nice."

They had never planned a funeral before; they didn't know anything. She couldn't think of any other options, and nobody offered her suggestions.

Her pastor recommended a funeral home and Jeff went alone. She wished she had gone with him, but she was physically and emotionally spent. Then Jeff went looking at cemetery plots by himself. She felt bad about that, too.

The funeral home provided their services free of charge, picking up Joshua's body from the hospital and supplying a small fabric-covered box that looked like a coffin from the set of a Dracula movie, but in miniature. The fabric, a white brocade, was the same material her wedding gown had been made from, making her smile and cringe simultaneously.

~ ~ ~

The burial was held on a perfect summer day. As they pulled up to the plot, Beth could see a small hole in the ground, the surrounding dirt covered with Astroturf, and two chairs side by side. Their pastor and Hank, from the funeral home, were there. She was wearing a maternity dress she had bought for Easter, something she felt pretty in, even today. Her hair was blowing in the wind and she felt like she was floating through some surreal movie. It was lonely with nobody there.

"Don't hug me because my milk came in, and I'm in too much pain," she said to her pastor. She had been shocked; it never occurred to her that milk would come after delivering a twenty-four-week-old baby. Nobody told her.

She sat next to Jeff and leaned into him, watching the pastor's lips move, unable to process the words. Hank made the sign of the cross on the top of the casket with dirt, and they left without watching Joshua being lowered into the ground. She was glad it was over. *Now I can move on,* she told herself, thinking she would be better shortly.

But it wasn't over, she couldn't move on, and one week later she found herself sobbing face down on the ground next to the mound of dirt covering Joshua's grave, with a burning desire to dig up her son's cold and lonely body.

Beth looked around and realized there were empty grave plots around Joshua's. Like Brittany, Joshua had been buried in a grandparent's plot, and one day he would share this space with that grandparent. But what about us? thought Beth. *When Jeff and I die, what if these plots are filled?* I want to be buried near my son.

She went immediately to the cemetery office and asked to purchase four plots next to Joshua's. At $900 each, Beth had to think twice. She and Jeff "didn't have a pot to piss in," financially speaking. But she didn't care. She signed a four-year financing agreement and went home that day the proud owner of "real estate" property.

Having Madeline to take care of gave Beth the will to get up each day, but she found tending to her daughter hindered her ability to grieve openly when she needed to. Beth had been seeing a counselor for depression during her pregnancy but stopped going one month before Josh died. Now, the depression deepened, and she found it increasingly difficult to face each day. She knew she needed help when she woke up one morning, unable to get out of bed, and asked herself, *Should I get up and go to the bathroom, or should I just wet the bed?* She went back to counseling and within two weeks was taking antidepressants. The medication didn't take away her grief; it merely helped her function.

Joshua had a birth certificate and a death certificate, and three weeks after he died, his social security card arrived in the mail; nobody told her it would come. "What the hell is this?!" she screamed at the mail.

After four weeks, she went back to her part-time job. Although some of her friends on the commuter train knew about Josh, many familiar faces didn't know. Before, she was pregnant; now she wasn't. What were they thinking? She felt self-conscious and awkward, uncomfortable with the idea of people talking about her.

People at work didn't avoid her, but didn't always bring the subject of Joshua up. They let her be the way she needed to be. There were days she could put on a smile and get through the day. But there were times when the look on her face said, "Don't talk to me, don't look at me, just leave me alone!" And they did.

She hated not knowing what Madeline was doing every moment and became obsessively paranoid something bad was going to happen to her only living child. She was almost waiting for Madeline to die next. Her paranoia grew, and she became so freaked out, she quit working after only one month.

Now Beth could stay home with Madeline, but things weren't perfect. She was plagued with feelings of guilt and blame, haunted by memories of not wanting Joshua in the beginning. She already felt she was a rotten mother to Madeline, and she wasn't any better after Josh's death. "Leave me alone!" she would scream at Madeline. She was afraid she was scarring the child, but couldn't control herself. *Madeline didn't ask for this. Look what I'm dragging her through,* Beth cried to herself.

She and Jeff coexisted. They didn't talk, they didn't fight, and they certainly didn't have sex. They were both grieving but didn't know how to help each other. She was still angry about the house she never wanted, a house that was a lot to take care of, a lot to clean, a lot to fix. She resented him for traveling and for not helping her more during the pregnancy. She partly blamed him for the loss of their son. And the memory of Joshua slipping through the birth canal and from her body was so vivid, it would be three months before she could even think about having intercourse again.

After a while, Jeff began to support Beth more. He supported her decision to quit working, but then their household expenses piled up: water, electric, food bills, mortgage. Beth's buying frenzy added to the problem; she was on a mission to find the perfect material thing to comfort her grieving soul. She bought any CD that had a special song that touched her heart; she had to have every angel she saw. "If Josh were here, I would have to buy things anyway," she rationalized. In August, they took a vacation, taking out a home equity loan to pay for the trip. They didn't care that it would add to their money problems. Their decisions were being guided by broken emotions.

In addition to counseling, Heidi had brought Beth to a place—
a circle of kindred hearts—where she was beginning to heal those broken emotions. But unlike Heidi, who had thrown herself headfirst into
a new pregnancy, Beth didn't know if she would ever have the courage
to face the uncertainty of a new pregnancy.

17

On a Sunday in March, I drop Alex off at her Sunday school class and join Al in our usual section, halfway back on the left side of church. Scanning the announcements, I see we'll be celebrating a baptism today. We've witnessed at least a dozen baptisms since last June, and each seems a little easier to swallow, but the first is burned in my memory.

It was Sunday morning, not even a week since our baby had died, and I had already begun asking the questions. *What went wrong? What kind of God are you?* We're good people and things like this aren't supposed to happen to good people. For twenty-seven years, I thought I was in control, that if I did everything right, everything would turn out okay. My beliefs about life might as well have followed my baby's spirit into the unknown, because they couldn't exist with me anymore.

I didn't expect to find the answers at church that June day—I wasn't sure the answers even existed—but Miranda's name would be offered during prayers, and I wanted to be there to hear it.

I looked around the crowded church and wondered if anyone knew what we had just gone through. I opened the bulletin to scan for Miranda's name, but found nothing. What I did see confirmed my worst fear: a baptism. I closed my eyes and took a deep breath, trying to keep my composure while the first reading began.

A chill radiated through my body as I listened to the story of a woman whose child had just died. The prophet Elijah took the boy into his arms and cried out to God to let the child's life come back into him. The boy came back to life, and Elijah gave him back to his mother.

Then the gospel told the story of Jesus as he passed a widow and the funeral procession of her only son. Jesus had compassion for her and told her not to weep. He then told the young man to rise, and the man did.

The intended message behind the stories was lost on me as I sat and wondered where Elijah and Jesus were when I could have used a miracle.

Pastor Needham looked over at us as he told the congregation the story about his neighbor's birth announcement and then a phone call from a couple in the hospital whose baby girl was stillborn. Al wrapped his arms around me as I cried, knowing everyone was probably wondering who the unlucky parents were.

When it was time for the baptism, my first instinct was to run out of the church, like in second grade at holy communion practice. I forgot to spit my gum out on the way in, and before I could run to the back to find a garbage can, Father Doody started talking. I was too afraid to get up in front of everybody to leave, so I stuck it in my hand. When it was my turn to go up to the altar, the gum had melted all over my hand—the hand that the wafer was supposed to go in—and up my sleeve. When Sister Barbara saw what I had done, she shook her head, pointed to the back, and told me to go clean myself up. I was certain that Father Doody was watching and all the kids were laughing.

"Are you going to be okay?" Al asked me, and before I could muster the courage to get up and leave, the family with the new baby was at the baptismal font, and I suddenly felt paralyzed. I forced the tears back and tried to be happy for this couple and their living baby, while what I really felt was angry and cheated. *It's not fair that Miranda had to be baptized in the middle of the night in a hospital recovery room. Why do they get to keep their baby when we didn't? Why us?* I asked over and over, digging into my purse, relieved to find a tissue still there from Miranda's memorial service the day before.

When the last notes of the organ finally trailed off, we made our way towards the back where the pastor was shaking hands. "Thank you for your sermon," I told him.

"How are you?" he asked.

"Good," we answered out of habit, but the wearied look on our faces told a different story.

Before we got out the doors, I saw my friend Sherry from the corner of my eye. She had lost a baby to miscarriage a few months earlier. At the time, I had little experience with miscarriage and didn't know what to say to her. Afraid of upsetting her if I asked about her loss, it was safer to say nothing at the time. Now, she was in my shoes. I knew she had seen me, but looked away. I headed for the doors, but something told me to stop. I turned around and walked over to her. "Sherry," I said, gently taking her arm, "I'm sorry about your miscarriage. I always wanted to tell you, but didn't know what to say."

She smiled with relief. "I'm so sorry for you, too. I didn't know what to say to you either." We gave each other a hug and promised to talk later.

~ ~ ~

Time seems to have sped up since last summer, the days are coming and going quicker than I can keep track, and now it's already the second Thursday of March. I can feel that my purpose in coming to support group meetings is no longer only about my grief; it's about helping others. Every month, a new face walks in the door. My friends and I look at each other with knowing. As newly bereaved parents tell their heartbreaking stories, we listen, understanding their pain, shock, and anger, and find ourselves offering words of encouragement and comfort, just as Dawn, who's not here tonight, had done for us so many months ago.

This month, after watching a video presentation of *When Bad Things Happen to Good People* by Rabbi Harold Kushner, based on his bestselling book, we move our chairs into a circle for open sharing time. The group is large tonight, but not too large for me to notice one of the new faces in the room. Her name is Wendy. She's tall with dark, short hair. Sitting next to her mom, who happens to be in town, Wendy tells us of her recent losses: Kelly, miscarried last August at thirteen weeks; then, just last month, she lost a second baby, David, at sixteen weeks after a premature delivery. After laboring, delivering, seeing, and then burying David, she hardly thinks of him as a miscarriage, but that's what most of the medical community still calls him. The hopelessness and pain in her life show, and Wendy sits through most of the meeting in silence.

Suddenly a woman sitting across the room from me begins to sob. We all watch and wait. "Rabbi Kushner doesn't believe God punishes us, but I feel so guilty. I just lost my baby girl, and a little voice in my head keeps whispering it's my fault. I had an abortion," she cries.

Beth, who's sitting next to her, puts her arms around the woman. "It's okay, you can talk about it."

The woman looks up and around the room not sure whether to talk or run, and several of us nod for her to go on. "I was young, just graduated from high school. I had a job and was planning to go to college in the fall when I found out I was pregnant. I didn't think I was capable of caring for a child, and my boyfriend didn't want a family. When I told him I wanted to carry the baby and give it up for adoption, he told me there was no way he would ever give up the child if I had it, so I had better get an abortion. When I missed work because of the morning sickness, my boss fired me. My parents, who didn't know about the pregnancy, thought I was a bum for lying around in bed with no job and kicked me out of the house. I had no job, no place to live, no support from my boyfriend or family. I never wanted the abortion, but I didn't know what to do. I felt trapped. I didn't know there were people, Christian groups, that would help me. I hated everyone, but most of all I hated myself."

She drops her head and cries again, and the room is silent. Beth squeezes her, and she takes a deep breath and continues. "I don't know why, but I always sensed the baby I aborted was a girl. A few years later, after I got married, my husband and I were so excited when I got pregnant with Melissa. Five months later, Melissa was born premature and didn't make it. The doctor called it incompetent cervix, and I read that a first trimester abortion could lead to incompetent cervix. Then my old boyfriend got married and had a little girl too, but he got to keep his baby. All I could think was I was being punished for that abortion. I took the life of that little baby, and God was doing the same to me. I don't really believe that, but sometimes I can't help but think it. I was afraid to let myself want the first baby, but I wanted Melissa more than life itself. I feel like I'm responsible for the deaths of two babies now, and I'm afraid I'll never have a little girl to love," she cries.

"You did the best you could," says Heidi. "You made the only choice you thought you had."

"Don't punish yourself for that," says Beth. "You need to forgive yourself."

Wiping the tears from her eyes, the woman looks at Beth with a grateful smile.

After the meeting, Wendy, the new woman who had two miscarriages, leaves with her mom before any of us can talk with her.

Beth invites Tracy, who's here without Jim, to the Omega with us. Beth is the kind of person who asks if you have anywhere to go for Thanksgiving and then invites you to her house, whether she knows you or not. She's the outgoing one in our group, making everyone feel welcome.

Tracy's eyes light up. "Sure, it's right by my house. They gave us balloons for Paul's funeral."

~ ~ ~

At the restaurant, Tony comes over to take our order. When he gets to Beth, she places her order for French toast with orange juice. Tony stops writing and looks at her.

"What?" she says looking up at him.

"No beer tonight?" he asks with a grin.

"No beer tonight," says Beth.

Tony laughs and heads for the kitchen shaking his head while Darlene leans over to explain to Tracy that Beth has been ordering beer with her French toast, until tonight.

I look at Beth, and then at Heidi, and then back at Beth. *Something's up*, I think to myself.

"Guess what?" asks Beth. "I'm pregnant!"

"Again?" I ask, my eyes popping open.

"Well, I didn't get my period this month, so I took another pregnancy test and it was positive. When I went to the doctor, I was shocked to see the tiny sac on the ultrasound screen. Jeff was out of town last month when I would have been ovulating, so my only conclusion is that it must have been an immaculate conception!" Everyone laughs. "The doctor told me maybe I didn't miscarry the first time after all, or maybe I miscarried a twin. I'd already talked myself into accepting Madeline as an only child. Now I'm trying to get used to the idea of a new baby all over again."

"How are you and Jeff getting along?" I ask Beth.

"You know, as angry as I was at him for a long time," says Beth, "our relationship has gotten better than before Josh died. It's the first time in our marriage that Jeff is actually taking care of me. Don't get me wrong, we still have a lot of issues, but we've been learning how to work together. I don't believe Josh died to save my marriage, but that was definitely a silver lining to a very gray cloud."

Darlene tells us she's been seeing three male cardinals sitting in the tree outside her balcony. "I think Nathan and Nicholas are visiting me," she says.

"Hey, I read in a book that many people have interesting experiences with red cardinals after someone they love dies," I say.

"Well, why are there three birds?" asks Heidi.

"I don't know, maybe the twins made a new friend." Everyone laughs.

18

In July of 1995, Darlene had been visiting her mom when sudden severe back pain doubled her over. She was halfway through her first pregnancy, twenty weeks, and hadn't experienced anything like this. Before she knew what was happening, amniotic fluid gushed from between her legs. She called Larry at work and her mother rushed her to the hospital. She was dilated to four centimeters when they stopped labor and performed an ultrasound.

"You're carrying twins," the doctor told her.

The news didn't come as a complete surprise to Darlene. She had suspected twins early on when her belly suddenly ballooned in the first trimester, she became terribly sick, and was sure she felt two babies moving inside. Her doctor had only detected one heartbeat at earlier appointments, though, and told her she would have to wait until her ultrasound at twenty-two weeks to find out.

That ultrasound came sooner than scheduled.

The monitor showed both babies alive and moving, facing each other with their hands and feet together. The hospital wasn't equipped to handle twenty-week-old infants, but the two closest high-risk hospitals wouldn't take her because she wasn't at least twenty-four weeks.

Darlene was told that if by a miracle they survived, the babies might be blind and hooked up to tubes for months, and even then there were no guarantees they would make it. Everything was happening so quickly, Darlene's head was spinning. "Don't do anything," she told them. "I don't want to keep my babies alive for my benefit only to have them die after suffering for months on end."

A nurse asked if they wanted a priest. Darlene didn't know why she would need a priest and, hesitant to wake someone up at midnight, said no. The staff told Darlene to call them when she felt pressure and they would come and check on her, leaving her and her mom to wait. Larry arrived shortly afterwards from work.

She was only dilated to five centimeters when the first baby, a boy, came out feet first and they rushed him out of the room. "Don't look at him," said Larry. "He looks like an alien." Darlene thought something must be wrong with the baby if he looked so strange. They did an ultrasound to check the other baby. There was no movement, no heartbeat; he was already gone. And he wasn't coming out. They hooked her up to Pitocin to induce contractions and everybody left the room.

She overheard the doctor talking to Larry and her mother in the hall. "Yes, don't worry about it, she can have more children. This is just a setback," the doctor assured. "She's got good hips, good bone structure."

The reality of the crisis had not yet hit Darlene. *Will everybody please stop crying!* she thought as she listened to Larry and her mother sobbing.

An hour later, the doctor reached in and pulled the second baby, another boy, out by his feet. Stillborn, he was immediately taken away, and Darlene was taken to recovery where a group of eight or so other women lay behind curtains. "I need to see my baby! I need to see my baby!" screamed a deaf woman from behind her curtain.

"Larry, go ask that husband to tell his wife to be quiet," said Darlene. Larry told her he couldn't do it. "Please, tell them our babies just died and we don't need to hear her screaming for her live baby."

"Darlene, I just can't."

~ ~ ~

It was 3:00 a.m., the fourth of July. A nurse opened the curtain and peaked her head in to check on Darlene. "Oh, by the way," she said, "your baby died over an hour ago." Then she left.

"What? Larry, go stop her!"

Larry brought the nurse back. "We didn't know our baby was still alive. Nobody told us!" said Darlene. "We assumed he couldn't breathe and died!"

"No, he was alive for a little over two hours. We were only watching him, watching his heart rate."

"Oh my God, Larry, he was alive."

Darlene sat helpless, too shocked, too numb to cry. Her son had lived two hours and she had missed every minute of it.

The nurse asked if they wanted to see him and Darlene told her no because she was afraid of looking at him after what Larry told her. Her mom and stepfather did, though, and came back crying.

They moved Darlene to the postpartum floor. "Where are your babies?" said the cleaning lady who walked in. "I want to see your babies."

Darlene's eyes flew open wide. "My babies died. I don't have babies."

"No, the other one, he's alive. Do you want to see your other one?"

"No, my babies died. I don't have any babies here."

"Yes, you're here on the baby floor, so your baby's here."

"No, I don't. I don't have babies!"

Darlene called the nurse. "This lady thinks I have a baby here. Are any of my babies alive?"

"No, they're both gone."

An hour later, Darlene told Larry to go get the nurse; she wanted to see her sons. The nurse brought in the firstborn wrapped in a blanket and set him on Darlene's lap, keeping her arm between him and his mother.

"Can I see the other one?" Darlene asked.

"You want to see the other one?"

"Yes."

"Well, he didn't live at all," said the nurse.

"I understand that, but can I see him?"

Twenty minutes later, the nurse came back holding the twins wrapped together in one blanket. She opened the blanket for Darlene and Larry to see. They didn't look like aliens. They were perfect and normal, just like full-grown babies, yet they were only ten inches long and weighed only ten ounces, and their skin was thin, almost transparent. After a few minutes, the nurse took them away.

~ ~ ~

Thirteen hours after being admitted to the hospital, Darlene was given a large manila envelope, told "This is some material for you when you go home," and was sent downstairs to be discharged.

"Did you name your child?" asked the clerk.

"Nathan Robert," Darlene answered. "Can I name the other one?"

"No, you're not allowed to name the other baby."

"Why?"

"Because he never lived and they don't get names if they've never lived. So we'll just have Nathan Robert and Baby B, okay?"

Darlene opened the envelope. Inside were two pamphlets: one about grieving, the other about miscarriage. Darlene was angry; at twenty weeks, she certainly didn't consider her babies miscarried— one was born alive, the other stillborn. She found a certificate with Nathan's footprints stamped in ink—none for Baby B—that measured from the tip of her pinky finger to her second knuckle—about one and a half inches. What she didn't expect to find were Polaroid pictures of her babies; nobody told her about the photos. The babies were photographed from the chest up, wrapped in a blanket. Arrows drawn in ink pointed this way and that to indicate the hospital got the two mixed up, writing the wrong names under each child. Nathan's cheek bones and ribs stuck out like a starving child's, but Baby B had round cheeks and a belly as if he had gotten more than his fair share of the food. Although a painful reminder, she thanked God because she knew without the photos she would quickly have forgotten her sons' faces.

~ ~ ~

Larry and Darlene decided to have their son's bodies cremated and were referred to a funeral home. "Why Baby B?" asked the funeral director.

"They wouldn't let us name him."

"Of course you can name him." He wrote a name and number down on a piece of paper. "Call this woman at the hospital and tell her you're going to name the child."

They went home, pulled out a baby name book and looked in the N section. "How about Nicholas?" she asked. "It's a great name. Nathan and Nicholas."

"Fine," answered Larry.

~ ~ ~

They had just moved into their new apartment and hadn't had time to decorate the nursery. The room was serving as a temporary office until the babies were born; what bedding and few baby items they had sat on the floor. But Darlene couldn't go in because she knew it was meant for them.

The apartment door was open to let the summer breeze in, and just outside stood the neighbors' one-year-old, crying for her father who had gone to take the garbage out. "Larry, please close the door. I can't bear to hear any children. Just close the door!"

"I'm sorry, but my wife's trying to sleep," Larry said to his new neighbor who had just returned. He didn't tell the neighbor his own children had just died.

Darlene stepped into the shower and turned on the water. She ran her hand down her stomach, now flat. And for the first time since losing her baby boys the night before, the tears came pouring out of her in waves.

~ ~ ~

Three days later, Larry's father sat them down and told them they had to get over it and move on.

"These were your grandsons, your only child's first children, and they're dead!" Darlene told him.

He ignored her remark. "The best thing for you to do is to sue the hospital. Both of you are piss poor. They didn't do anything to save these babies. Sue them and then live the rest of your lives happily."

"You know, right now I couldn't care less how little money we have or how much we could have," said Darlene. "I'd rather have them back more than anything. We're not going to sue anybody because they're going to bring up every little thing I did or didn't do, and you know I drank Diet Coke—I think I drank two that day. They could say I drank two Diet Cokes and that's what brought on my labor. I am not going to be dragged through the mud and keep this as fresh in my head for the next two years as it is now!"

"But think of the money!"

"I don't give a shit about the money. I can't go on with this conversation. Larry take me home."

~ ~ ~

Larry went back to work, and every night for a week he came home to find Darlene where he left her: sitting on the couch in her pajamas with the blinds closed, crying and holding a tiny sweater and some blankets his grandmother had made during the pregnancy, milk leaking from her breasts. They didn't tell her to expect milk. When she asked her doctor what to do about her engorged breasts, he told her to sit in a bath of warm water to help some of the milk come out and relieve it. What it did for her was keep the milk leaking out for the next year.

At night, she slept with her head at the foot of the bed for a better view in case her babies came into the room through the door. Larry thought she was going crazy.

Darlene didn't know what Larry felt. They had been married only nine days when her water broke, engaged only five months before that, and had spent a good part of their courtship apart while Larry was away at college. They were still learning about each other when their lives were torn apart. The twenty-year-old didn't know how to talk to her new husband about the emotions they were both facing.

Although unplanned, the pregnancy hadn't come as a complete surprise to them. He had been excited about the pregnancy; she knew that much. He was an only child and his entire family could fit around one table. But Darlene's mom was one of eight children, and Darlene's aunt had seven of her own children. At holiday gatherings, her extended family took up the entire house. He liked that and told her he wanted a large family; she wanted the same.

~ ~ ~

Six weeks went by and friends were telling her she had to get normal again. "You gotta get back to yourself. You're not eating. You're not joking around. You're not going out. You're not doing anything." Darlene didn't want to do anything, but she started to think they were right. *Maybe I'm not normal. Maybe I'm supposed to be over this after six weeks. Maybe I'm supposed to get on with my life,* she thought. This is crazy. *I can't just sit at home and lose my mind. There've got to be books on this.*

She went down to the apartment manager's office to pay the rent and asked where the local public library was. "I'll show you where the library is," said a hugely pregnant woman behind her. "I'm usually never down here, but I'm on maternity leave."

"Oh. So am I," said Darlene.

"You are? Where's your baby?"

"Well, unfortunately they died. I had twins."

The woman looked at her and nodded with knowing. "I'm sorry. I'm a bereavement counselor."

"You are?"

"Yes, but since I'm on maternity leave, let me give you the name of a lady at another hospital. Her name is Pat Vaci. You have to call her. She's wonderful. They have a support group. You'll meet other people who have gone through this."

"That's why I'm going to the library, to look for books about loss."

"Yeah, there are books, but go see these people and hear what they have to say, and let it off your chest."

Darlene thanked the woman, found some books at the library, and came home and called Pat.

"I just lost them in July. I don't know what to do, I'm losing my mind," Darlene cried over the phone. "I met this lady and she told me to call you."

"I want you to come to our meeting," said Pat. "It's in two days."

Darlene came to that meeting and was welcomed with open arms. It wasn't long before she was spending her days commiserating with Heidi and Beth.

19

"That's it, I'm through!" I yell, sitting on the toilet in the bathroom, looking down into a bowl now turned red. I've gotten my period—again. I'm tired of taking my temperature every morning. I'm tired of charting mucus every day. I'm tired of spending twenty-five dollars on ovulation predictor kits. I'm too stressed-out to worry about getting pregnant now that we're preparing for our upcoming move into a new house: a two-story colonial with four bedrooms that seems too big for a family of three.

For a distraction, I take Alex on a sunny spring day to visit the park in the new neighborhood we'll soon be moving to. It's a beautiful little park, with long stretches of grass and trees and a playground with a miniature train. "Miranda!" My ears and eyes perk up. "Miranda, come here," calls a mother. A little girl comes running from the slide. This is the first Miranda I've seen, living. *That's nice,* I think. But the more her mother calls her name, the more I'm reminded that I'll never be able to. *That's my daughter's name, but she's dead,* I want to tell the woman. Finally, I can't stand it anymore and pull Alex to the car, ignoring her cries to stay longer, hoping this little girl with my dead child's name isn't one of my new neighbors.

~ ~ ~

On an April evening, with the day's last rays of sunlight stream-
ing down through stained-glass windows, Pat opens the spring memorial service with words from "A Prayer for Spring" by Janis Heil. "Life
has dared to go on around me. And as I recover from the insult of life's
continuance, I readjust my focus to include recovery and growth as a
possibility in my future. Give me strength to break out of the cocoon
of my grief. But may I never forget it as the place where I grew my
wings, becoming a new person because of my loss."

I realize I am slowly becoming that new person, like it or not.
I appreciate more deeply things in my life I have always taken for
granted: my husband, daughter, health, home, my own life. Sometimes
I sit staring at Al and Alex and try to imagine what my life would be
like if one of them wasn't here. Or what if one of us faced a serious illness? I look around my house and wonder what I would do if I did-
n't have a home at all. And what if I wasn't here anymore and Al had
to raise Alex without me?

The new person I am is more conscious of life. The first time
I found a spider in the bathroom after Miranda died, I couldn't bring
myself to kill it as I usually would have. I went all the way downstairs
to the kitchen to get a container, went back up the stairs to the bathroom, caught the spider, went back downstairs carrying the spider, and
let it go in the backyard. Even though spiders creep me out, I now have
an entire colony of them in the backyard.

The old me used to get so agitated when things didn't go perfectly, it would sometimes take hours for my mood to recover. I realized this had changed the first time I came home with a bag of food
from a local fast food drive-thru and discovered they had neglected to
put the cheese on my cheeseburger—a cardinal sin to this serious
cheese lover. In the past, this mistake would have me fuming almost to
the point of refusing to eat, but not before making an angry phone call
to the manager. Now, I no longer get bent out of shape, but simply
shrug, assume they were training a new employee, and tell myself I'm
better off without the cheese.

I'm also more likely to reach out to other people who need a friend or a compassionate listener. Last month, our pastor told us about a couple in our congregation who had recently lost the infant twin sister of their healthy new baby girl and asked if we would offer support, adding that they were already expecting our call. We couldn't say no. After Miranda's memorial service last summer, we had told him to call on us if another family ever lost a baby. But now I realized living through grief and being qualified to help someone through it are two entirely different things, and I wondered what I would say.

I pulled out the church phone directory looking for the family, wondering if our paths had ever unknowingly crossed. Recognizing them and their two older daughters, I took a deep breath and dialed their number. Her husband answered and I told him who I was, how sorry I was, and asked how he was doing, not really knowing what to say to a man, but knowing he was grieving as much as his wife and knowing many people were only going to ask about her.

When his wife got on the phone, I went through the same rehearsed introduction. Like her husband, she seemed to appreciate my call.

"When our baby died, I was in shock and was angry that my healthy baby died so suddenly from an accident," I told her. She was sad too, but knew early on that her second twin's chances of survival weren't good. She had time to prepare.

"I battled with loneliness and depression for a long time," I told her. She was too busy taking care of a newborn and two other children to feel those emotions, she said.

"I still have a hard time with baptisms and music. Do you have that problem too?" No, not really, she told me, because they still had the other baby.

"I found a lot of comfort from a support group. It's helped me a lot, and I've made some really close friends." She said she and her husband knew of a support group for parents of multiples, but didn't know if they would go.

I hung up feeling like I didn't help her at all. In fact, she didn't seem to need help. Yet, I knew from my support group that, regardless of how many other children a couple had, losing a twin could be devastating, the living child being a constant reminder of the missing child that should be sharing bedrooms and birthdays and walking hand in hand through life with the one still here.

Nevertheless, I took over a loaf of banana bread and told her I would talk with her again. After church services each week, Al and I ask how they are, make small talk, and smile at their twin without a twin.

Now, as I look around the chapel, I wonder if any of these families are here to remember the loss of one of their twins. Pat announces that each family will receive a memorial keepsake, and everyone takes turns getting up and walking to the front where Heidi and Beth are passing out soft, white lamb pins. Parents of living children collect photos, finger paintings, school poems; bereaved parents collect memorial service keepsakes and candles, and bulletin inserts from church.

One week earlier, on Easter Sunday, I had come home from church with my bulletin insert. As I pulled down Miranda's box from my closet shelf, I realized that in twenty years I would have a box full of bulletin inserts, all printed with the same words: *In Memory of Miranda Novak*. I didn't need a piece of paper to remind me of her. I put the box back on the shelf, went downstairs, and tossed the insert into the recycling bin, deciding that memorial keepsakes would be one of the few things I would save from now on.

The highlight of the spring service is the dedication of the memorial quilt, hanging on the wall, beautifully framed. The six of us—Dawn, Heidi, Beth, Darlene, Tracy, and I—stand with our arms around each other, smiling and sniffling, appreciating the meaning, beauty, and uniqueness of each square. Some are cross-stitched, others embroidered, a few handwritten, with names, dates, poetry, or messages of love.

My heart beats fast until my eyes come to rest on Miranda's square—a project I spent an entire week arranging, rearranging, cutting, and gluing until it was just right: a baby angel with a wreath of bows and flowers in her hair, kneeling against a purple pansy, words written with lavender fabric paint: *Miranda Blair Novak, June 20, 1995, Forever in Our Hearts.*

Wendy, the new woman who joined our group the previous month, stands alone behind us; her two miscarried babies will have to wait until next year's quilt. Beth turns around and pulls Wendy in with us, our arms surrounding her. Just as the quilt has brought each of our children together, our children have brought each of us together. Despite the circumstances, we leave this day grateful for the friendships we've made and now treasure.

On the way out the door, I wave to Tracy and Jim as they pull out of the parking lot. *I thought for sure Paul's quilt square would have a monkey on it,* I think to myself, grinning. One of these days I'd really like to meet that monkey.

20

There was no doubt in her mind: Tracy wanted children. But her first husband, reluctant to make that commitment, convinced her to wait five years. Those years came and went, and Tracy realized she had been living on a false promise. It was the breaking point in a marriage doomed from the start.

When Tracy met Jim, they were in their mid-thirties, and as they began to talk about marriage, children were always a part of the plan as well. Jim was sincere in his desire to be a father, and soon after the wedding, they began efforts to conceive. "This is a really good day to try, Jim," Tracy would say with a grin. Their lovemaking was planned and calculated. Tracy had been tracking her menstrual cycle and taking her temperature and knew, technically, conception should be happening. "This would be a really good day, Jim," Tracy would say the next month, and the next, and the next. She teetered between the joy of anticipation and the heartbreak of disappointment.

After six months with no pregnancy, Tracy's doctor shot dye through Tracy's fallopian tubes to look for blockages—a hysterosalpingogram. Everything was clear. One month later, he took a cervical biopsy to check for cellular changes. The results were inconclusive.

A few weeks later, when her period didn't come, she got up early and took the pregnancy test that had been sitting in the bathroom. "Brandy!" she whispered, trying not to wake Jim. The Chesapeake Bay Retriever poked her head around the corner, wondering what could be so important; she knew it wasn't time for her walk. "Guess what?" she whispered, the dog's ears perking up. "We're going to have a baby! Don't tell Jim. This is our little secret." She patted the dog on the head and quietly snuck out of the house, heading for a nearby hospital where she worked as a medical technologist.

When she came home that day, she baked a small cake, carefully picking out all the pink and blue sprinkles from the bottle and placing them on the top. When Jim, a high school math teacher, got home from school that afternoon, Tracy put the cake down in front of him, trying to hide the excitement. "Jim, guess what?"

He looked down at the cake and then up at her with a blank look on his face. "What?"

"Jim! We're going to have a baby!"

"Ohhhhh. I was wondering when you were going to take that test."

It was 1995, and Tracy's baby was due in November. Her pregnancy was a dream come true, and she enjoyed every minute of it. Her full-time job kept her busy while the pregnancy sailed along, and every kick brought Tracy's hand to her belly and a smile to her face. Jim, who couldn't carry a tune to save his life, often put his hand on Tracy's growing abdomen and sang the tune to the song "How much is that doggy in the window?" changing the words to "What sex is that baby in the belly?" She and Jim were ready in every sense to have this baby: financially, emotionally, mentally, spiritually.

November quickly arrived, and by her due date, she had begun to dilate and her cervix was thinning. *Is this going to be the day?* she asked herself every morning.

The following Monday, when she woke up still pregnant, still not in labor, the tears poured out. *Now I have to go to work and everyone's going to say, "Are you still here?"* She was busy that day and worked through lunch, occasionally feeling a kick or jab from the baby. Relaxing in the bathtub that evening, she began contracting at regular intervals and was soon on her way to the hospital.

"Oh, this is it!" said the nurses on the way to the birthing room. "Change into this gown and jump up on the bed. We're going to have a little look." They put the doppler monitor on her belly and waited for the baby's heartbeat. The empty static of the monitor echoed through the room. They tried the bedside ultrasound. The two nurses looked at each other. "We're going to get another machine." Tracy read the look on both their faces.

"That baby is dead!" Tracy shouted. "That baby is dead! We've always found the heartbeat right away, even in the very beginning!"

The doctor came in aware of the situation. "We're going to take you down to ultrasound," he said.

"Don't even bother," Tracy told him. "The baby's not alive."

The doctor looked at her intently. He reached over and turned the monitor off. "We're going to leave you alone and give you some time to sort things out." Everyone quietly filed out of the room as Jim and Tracy sat in shock.

This is not happening. This must be a dream. It was like getting hit from behind; they didn't see it coming. *This is not supposed to happen.* She knew miscarriage was common and had heard of people losing babies before term, but to think she was going to have this baby, this full-term baby, and then find out it was dead was horrifying. She and Jim tried to process what was happening but were distraught and couldn't think clearly. When the doctor came back in the room, Tracy told him to "get this baby out of me. I don't want it in me. Just get it out." Jim asked if she could have a c-section, but the doctor told him no because Tracy wasn't at risk.

She called her father, who lived in California, and told him the baby had died. He was devastated and told her he was going to catch the next plane out to Chicago. Tracy told him not to bother.

Her mother, who lived nearby, arrived shortly with Reverend Dan, a family friend and minister who had performed Tracy and Jim's wedding ceremony.

Tracy hadn't slept well the night before and was exhausted. The doctor stopped her labor so she could get some rest. It didn't matter; she didn't rest that night. The darkness and quiet of the room was agonizing. As Jim slept beside her bed, her mind raced, yet the minutes seemed like hours. It seemed like morning would never come.

Both of their families came the next day, and Tracy's dad arrived from California despite his daughter's advice. Father Joe, the pastor from their church, waited with everyone outside Tracy's room while she and Jim prepared for labor. Stepping into the shower to clear her head, she readied herself mentally for the hardest thing she would ever have to do.

Tracy declined pain medication; she didn't know if she would ever get another chance to deliver a baby and wanted to feel every contraction. But the Pitocin brought labor on so hard and strong, she couldn't handle it anymore and asked for an epidural. Now numbed from the waist down, she pushed for two hours trying to deliver a baby that couldn't help her, and the doctor had to use forceps to pull the baby out.

"It's a boy."

Despite the mark on his face left by the forceps, he was a beautiful baby, perfect in every way. Tracy was suddenly so happy. It was strange, but even though he was dead, she was proud of him. The nurse spread a towel over Tracy and the doctor laid the wet, warm baby boy on Tracy's chest.

Tracy's blood pressure was dropping and she began to fade out. The nurse took the baby, cleaned him, and wrapped him up, and when Tracy stabilized, the nurse handed him back to her. She sat looking down at him, rocking quietly. Tracy and Jim passed their son back and forth while the nurse snapped pictures. Family filed in and took turns holding their grandson and nephew. The room was wall-to-wall with people, clearly breaking hospital regulations, but it didn't matter.

The nursing staff tried to be compassionate, but it was obvious to Tracy they were uncomfortable and ill-prepared to deal with the situation. She didn't know what to do either, but was comforted by the presence of her family. One by one, she looked into the faces of her loved ones, wondering what they must be thinking as they held this tiny, perfect dead baby in their arms. She watched her younger brother, the sensitive emotional one, as he stood by her side, never holding the baby. Perhaps it was too much for him.

They had a boy's name picked out, but decided to save that name in case they ever had another son. For this child they chose the name Paul Matthew, "an appropriate and fitting name for a soul standing at the pearly gates," according to Jim. "Besides," he pointed out, "we could never have given him the name Paul if he had lived, because his initials would have been *PU* and kids are so cruel. He should be safe from teasing because angels would never make fun of another angel's name."

Their friend, Reverend Dan, gave a short service, delivering a touching eulogy, and then Father Joe, dear sweet man, was so flustered during the baptism he called the baby Paul Margaret by mistake.

Tracy had delivered at the hospital where she worked and the next day called down to her department and asked them not to come to her room. Decisions were made for her while she sat alone in her bed, numb. An autopsy was performed and Paul's body was taken to a funeral home and prepared for burial.

"Oh how wonderful!" said the department store clerk as she wrapped a christening gown, cap, and booties that Tracy's mom had picked out.

"No, not really," answered Tracy's mom, fighting back the tears. "We're burying my grandson in that."

Tracy's mom was fighting a double battle. All these years she had hidden the grief of losing her firstborn child in stillbirth. Tracy and her two younger brothers were never told about their older sister, and Tracy knew only after finding the death certificate while recently going through her mother's papers. Now her divorced parents were grieving for their lost grandchild and silently reliving their worst nightmare through Tracy.

Jim, along with Tracy's dad and brother, went to pick out a casket, taking with him some things he had gathered to be buried with Paul: the baseball bat Tracy's dad had brought from California with Paul's name etched in it and the baseball booties he had sent during the pregnancy, a picture of Tracy pregnant, a picture of the house Paul would have grown up in, a family wedding picture, the rosary from Tracy's first communion, and a book in which they wrote a letter to their son:

> *To our beloved son, Paul Matthew,*
>
> *From the day you were conceived, we waited with joyful anticipation for the day we could meet you. Not a day went by without a loving pat to Mommy's belly, a silly song or a softly spoken word to you, our dear baby. As your birth approached, the excitement heightened. We made so many plans, all including you. Our lives changed forever with the news that you had died. Your birth was a bittersweet one. Mommy delivered you into Daddy's arms. We, your family and friends, marveled at you, beautiful and perfect son, grandson, nephew, and cousin. With your journey on earth done before it started, we put our trust in the Lord. Look down on us from heaven. Know that you will always be in our hearts. We are comforted to know that we will be together again some day. We love you to the moon and back. With eternal love, Mommy and Daddy*

Since they weren't having a wake, Jim took a picture of Paul in the casket.

Tracy, kept in the hospital another day because of heavy bleeding, finally allowed visitors in her room. As she showed her coworkers the Polaroid pictures of Paul, she couldn't imagine what they were thinking. People wanted to be supportive, but didn't know how to react; she was in such a state of shock she wasn't paying attention to what they were saying to her anyway. All she could think of was Paul, that he was so beautiful—her perfect angel.

The hospital social worker never came to see Tracy, but the nurse gave her a small folder to take with her, containing a pamphlet about a bereavement group at the hospital; a certificate titled "Memories," listing Paul's birth statistics, and his footprints stamped in ink; the little knit cap with a blue ball; a tiny gold ring; and photos taken by the nurse—a few of Paul alone, some with his parents. In every picture, Jim's face beamed like any proud father's, concealing the pain of the moment. But the devastation on Tracy's face confirmed the truth of a breaking heart and unspeakable grief.

At home, the nursery that had patiently awaited the arrival of its tiny occupant remained untouched, the door left open. For months Tracy had lovingly prepared this special room for her new baby; it was unreal to her that it was occupied now only by stuffed animals, sympathy cards placed carefully like a shrine, and baby gifts in the closet. Tracy hadn't wanted a baby shower, and her mom didn't believe in them either, probably because of losing her own firstborn, yet her mom had surprised Tracy with a small shower anyway, inviting a few friends to a restaurant. It would be a long time before Tracy would be able to attend a baby shower. Almost as difficult would be the sight of pregnant women, which would haunt Tracy for years to come.

~ ~ ~

It was 9:30 p.m. the night before the burial when Tracy told Jim she wanted to release balloons at the cemetery the next morning. "But where are we going to get helium balloons this late?" she asked Jim.

"I have an idea," he said. He got in the car and drove down the street to the Omega restaurant. When he walked in, his face wore the stress of the past few days: he hadn't shaven; his clothes were disheveled;

he looked like he lived on the street. The manager surveyed Jim from across the room and walked over with concern. "Can I give you a meal?" he asked. Jim smiled.

"We lost our son and we're burying him tomorrow. Would you mind giving us a few balloons?"

Tracy laughed when Jim told her what had happened, and soon Jim was laughing with her. It was the first time in days that they had laughed, and for a moment they felt normal. After that, whenever Jim skipped a few days of shaving, Tracy teased, "You're looking like you need a free meal, Jim."

At 3:00 a.m., she woke up bleeding so heavily she had to send Jim out again, this time to the pharmacy for more sanitary pads.

The next morning, cold, gray, and miserable, the hearse drove by their house on the way to the cemetery, Tracy and Jim pulling out behind it. She later wished they had simply put Paul's casket in their car and driven it themselves, although she didn't know if there was a law against it.

Family and friends, some from childhood, gathered in the cemetery chapel. Many had taken the day off work. Someone from the funeral home said a few words, and then Jim, her dad and brothers, and the other men went to the gravesite to watch Paul's casket being lowered into the ground. They didn't think Tracy should go to the gravesite, so she waited in the chapel with her mom and the women. Her milk had just come in. She was in a lot of pain and kept her distance from everyone.

She thought about her phone call the day before to Gina, one of her dearest friends, to tell her of the arrangements. "I appreciate you inviting me, but that's kind of just for family. I'm not going to come." Tracy told Gina she understood, but was devastated just the same. Gina sent some books on perinatal loss and checked in with her often, though, and they remained close friends.

After the burial, the family gathered in a private room at a local pizza place. Papa's had become a family tradition; it was where Tracy's mom had met Jim's family for the first time, and after their wedding, everyone had headed to Papa's for a big party. Now, Tracy's dad brought a bat, identical to the one buried with Paul, and the restaurant put it in a display case on the wall. They brought home a napkin full of cherry tomatoes for Brandy, their vegetable-loving dog—the only "baby" Tracy was able to take care of now.

A few days after the burial, Jim took Tracy to the children's section of the cemetery so she could see where Paul's grave was. She was appalled to find that someone had taken the buds off the roses until they discovered resident deer were eating the flowers. She left a small decorated Christmas tree by his grave so she could find it again until his headstone was in place.

~ ~ ~

Replaying the events of Paul's birth became an exhausting and all-consuming task, and Tracy turned to a yellow legal pad to get the thoughts out of her head. The words—scribbled details combined with raw emotion—were anything but fine prose, but it gave her temporary relief and the reassurance that she wouldn't forget the emotions and events of her darkest days. The more she wrote, the more clear the events became. She remembered the movie that night—the night before he died—and the baby's unusual activity after a loud scene. *Might that have been the end?*

She was used to having control over things in her life and everything had been planned out so carefully. She struggled now at being out of control, yet there was nothing she could do. Well-meaning people told her, "God never gives you more than you can handle." She didn't want to believe God was dishing it out. She didn't blame anyone. She was just angry things didn't turn out the way they were supposed to.

Jim went back to work, Tracy was left home without a baby, and as the shock began to wear off, depression set in. She called the number for the pregnancy loss support group the nurse had given her. "We don't have that group anymore," a woman told her. "They stopped meeting a long time ago." Tracy was in despair. Who could she turn to now? Who knew what she was going through?

A coworker of Jim's, who had lost a baby the previous year, told them about a pregnancy loss support group that had helped them. The facilitator's name was Pat Vaci.

Tracy called Pat within a week of coming home from the hospital, encouraged that there was a monthly group she could turn to for help, but the next meeting was a Christmas memorial service. She would have to wait until January for a regular group meeting. She marked her calendar for the December memorial; it was better than nothing.

~ ~ ~

Outside, it seemed to rain every day that November, mirroring the tear drops pouring from inside Tracy. The few times she laughed after Paul died, she wondered if she was dishonoring her child by feeling good and rebelling against grief's tight hold.

Jim seemed better. He was teaching. He was functioning. He wanted her to be better too, but she wasn't getting there. It was hard for him to see her so sad every day when he got home. "I want my old wife back," he told her. Tracy looked at him.

"I will never be the same. Good or bad, losing Paul changed me, changed my life like nothing else ever can or ever will again."

Emotionally, there wasn't a lower place to be, thinking she couldn't go on another day. She never thought she was going to kill herself, but she didn't feel safe anymore and whenever driving became afraid someone was going to crash into her. It didn't matter to her if she died now anyway because life as she knew it was over. This was her new life, her new reality. Her life was categorized into two parts: life before Paul and life after Paul.

Occasionally Tracy would go into the nursery, a peaceful place for her, and rearrange the cards on top of Paul's dresser. During one of her visits to her son's empty room, she found the breast pump and milk storage bags she had bought from a specialty baby store during her pregnancy, eager to breastfeed her baby. When she went back to the store to return them, the clerk looked at the receipt. "Well, it's past thirty days, we can't accept returns after thirty days," she said handing it back to Tracy.

"Well, I have a dead baby!" Tracy snapped. "My baby died and I don't intend to use this right now!" The clerk's face went pale and she rushed off to get the manager.

"It's okay, we'll give you your money back," said the manager. Tracy was furious. She hoped they were shocked and she hoped they felt bad.

~ ~ ~

Tracy had so little of Paul, she was grasping for anything she could get and went to the doctor's office to ask for the tracing of his movement from a nonstress test. She wanted the last one because it was the closest she could get to his last moments, the few days before his death. Something wasn't right; they wouldn't give it to her, and she began to wonder if maybe that test signaled the beginning of the end to Paul's life. They instead gave her the one from the previous week. Tracy didn't push the issue. She knew she couldn't bring Paul back, and there was nothing she could have done to prevent Paul's death.

The results of Paul's gross autopsy had come back inconclusive. Everything was normal. No reason. The report went into great detail, even describing the brain. *Oh my God, they cut open his head. She suddenly felt sick. Why did we have this done?* she cried. *It was only his shell, Tracy,* she had to remind herself. *You needed to know.* All they could tell her was Paul had died sometime Monday, the day she went into labor. But nothing else. Maybe the due date was wrong, like Tracy had suspected. She wracked her brains to calculate dates again. Maybe he had been allowed to go too long in utero. *Should I have been induced earlier?* Yet, his weight was just under eight pounds; he was an average-sized baby. She was relieved there was no genetic reason, no abnormality that should repeat itself with another pregnancy.

Thanksgiving was approaching and Tracy and Jim felt they had nothing to be thankful for. Nobody felt like celebrating much less cooking, so instead of the usual feast her mom cooked every year, they went to a hotel restaurant with Tracy's family.

As Christmas approached, Tracy went through the motions of gift shopping and card sending. Only, this year, the card contained a note about the loss of a son, so dearly loved, so eagerly anticipated, and sorely missed.

~ ~ ~

Pat Vaci met Tracy and Jim at the door and welcomed them in. It was the Christmas memorial service, the only way they could think of to spend Christmas with Paul in a special way. Surrounded by strangers, they headed for the back of the room. She was unsettled by the presence of a nearby toddler, but the parents had just lost twins. She understood. After the readings and songs, Tracy took her turn hanging a chubby Dreamsicle angel baby ornament on the tree for Paul. They went through a lot of tissues, but so did everyone else and they realized it was okay. Being here, with these people, brought them the comfort they were hoping for.

Christmas evening, Tracy and Jim had dinner at her mom's, but she struggled to be near her sister-in-law who was bursting with her thirty-nine-week pregnancy, and Jim took her home early. She still clung to month-old feelings of resentment because her sister-in-law, eight months pregnant at the time, hadn't come to the hospital when Tracy delivered Paul. *How could she have come?* Tracy later realized. *It would have been too upsetting for her to see me grieving over my dead baby and too upsetting for me to see her so pregnant.*

A few nights later, Tracy and her mom attended mass at a local church to celebrate Feast of the Holy Innocents. Traditionally a remembrance of the babies slain at the hands of Herod in his mad search for the baby Jesus, the mass took on a broader meaning for families whose children had died in a state of innocence. The church was full. Tracy lit a candle in memory of Paul and urged her mom to light a candle for her long ago stillborn daughter, whose name, Tracy learned, was Gail.

Spending the remainder of Jim's Christmas break in Canada, accompanied by the tree-top monkey, one night they went out for a walk on the golf course, writing Paul's name in big letters in the snow with their feet. When they came inside, they received the call from Tracy's brother that he and his wife had just delivered their new daughter, Hannah. "Oh, that's really great," she told her brother, trying to sound convincing. But deep in her heart, Tracy was devastated.

Upon returning home, they went to the hospital and as Tracy held Hannah, both she and Jim cried. Inside their hearts, a battle was waging between joy and despair. Still, it felt good to hold a newborn, even someone else's. After the baby came home from the hospital, she and Jim went to her brother's house to see her again, and this time everybody cried.

When Tracy's sister-in-law went back to work, Hannah was taken to a daycare center. But she wasn't adjusting well and suddenly her parents found themselves needing emergency child care. They called Tracy and she agreed to help. But, the baby cried and cried and wouldn't take a bottle, and by the end of the day Tracy cried, too. *Maybe God knew what he was doing. Maybe I wasn't meant to be a mother because I don't know how to be a mother! I can't do anything right!* Tracy told them she couldn't watch Hannah anymore.

Just as her anger began to well up inside, her doctor recommended the book *When Bad Things Happen to Good People* by Rabbi Harold Kushner, a bereaved parent himself. Rabbi Kushner's take on life was that losing a child is one of those unfair things that happen, that God would not intend for it to happen to you, and it wasn't for a purpose, and it wasn't to see how you would handle it, or to burden you, or to test your faith. God weeps with you. You can lean on Him or you can be angry with Him, and it's okay because He can handle it. Reading this book helped squelch her anger before she directed it towards God.

~ ~ ~

Tracy was starting to face the days and trying to function without being totally consumed with Paul's death. She felt better physically and her energy was returning. But she didn't feel like she was making any progress being home alone, and after the busyness of the holidays, she didn't know what to do with herself. She was getting this vibe from people: okay, it's been long enough, time to move on.

Tracy had only planned on going back to work part time after the baby was born, but now with no baby to love and care for, she was back full time. Her coworkers were supportive, but she felt the pressure to function at a high level and she wasn't ready to do that. A few people pulled her aside and asked her to talk about Paul and what had happened. Tracy learned that while she was on leave, her department manager arranged a memorial service at work for Paul and read some words in his honor. Tracy was touched that this woman, who rarely displayed compassion, had acknowledged Paul in such a special way.

Tracy immersed herself in work and taking care of the dog, often taking long walks just to be with herself. She felt alone most of the time, except when she talked with other people who had experienced loss. Tracy read and read and read; she couldn't get her hands on enough stories about other people who had lost babies, and although the stories sometimes made her sad, she needed to face the pain head on.

She also obsessed about getting pregnant again; she needed to have another baby. In her mind, that was how she was going to heal. Both she and Jim wanted to move to a more positive place instead of wallowing in grief, to move forward with their life together. She was taking her temperature again and her cycles were regular, but nothing was happening, and she and Jim were growing increasingly frustrated.

~ ~ ~

Tracy lived for the second Thursday of the month: support group night. We helped validate her feelings and validated Paul as her son. "People who haven't lost a child have no idea. They just have no idea. That person is still your baby, still part of your family," she said at her first meeting. She was angry that people didn't know how devastated she was, how all-consuming the grieving process was.

For the first few months, she showed up with one thing to say, something she had been holding onto that she had to get out. Often, it was something somebody had said to her, words she knew were meant to be helpful, but instead hurt her to the core. There were no other places to go and say these things. Other people tried to help her, but the support group was the one safe place where she knew she could say anything without being judged or thought crazy, where everyone in the room understood. The group could handle the hurt and anger she had been holding onto. Once she got it out, she was done with it and could finally let it go.

Tracy left meetings feeling emotionally drained, but she had found a way to release the negative emotions and thoughts. The tears were the vehicle in which they traveled, and our support group was the fuel.

21

Nearly one year ago I asked the question, *How do I survive the death of my baby?* The answer came to me not so much in words, although the books I had chosen to read gently guided me towards a place of healing. The answer came in less direct form: a phone call from a cousin; a card from my mom; a lunch invitation from a friend; the Share support group; Omega restaurant rendezvous with my six friends whom I fondly think of as *The Good Grief Club.* Even a sympathetic smile from someone conveying the message "I still remember" was enough to get me through each day, one at a time, with my sanity and hope still in tact. Every gesture from another human being was like a refueling jet, pulling up alongside me, filling my soul up just before I nosedived and crashed to the ground. As the pain and anger subside, one question still remains. What was it all for?

In the midst of my search for answers to the meaning of Miranda's short life, my mom invites me to go with her to see a man named Edward. He is a medium, a person who receives communication from spirits of loved ones on the other side, and has traveled from Canada to the home of a dear family friend, Sher—a psychologist, lecturer, author, and healer. I've been told not to have expectations, especially regarding someone who has recently died or "crossed over."

I understand, but there is only one reason I'm here, only one person I want to hear from.

As I follow Edward, a middle-aged man wearing a button-down shirt, sweat pants, and slippers—a casual medium—down the hall, I remember the psychic I had previously visited. Although she didn't claim to be able to communicate with my loved ones, I had hoped for some bit of information about Miranda and couldn't help but feel disappointed that it didn't happen. Her house predictions ended up being quite accurate, though. Our new house had everything she said it would except for the bay window. She was also right about me not getting a fence, and my dog stayed put with my parents where he had room to run.

Edward leads me into a main floor bedroom, and we sit in two folding chairs facing each other. He closes his eyes and begins by telling me about my past lives. Under normal circumstances the history lover in me would find the information quite fascinating: something about me being a performer in eighteenth-century Spain, but not wanting to be a mother, I had aborted several babies. This last piece of information I find hard to swallow, considering I've come here for the sole purpose of communicating with my much-loved, much-wanted baby girl.

My heart beats faster as each of my sixty minutes ticks by without mention of the presence of a baby, and as the cassette tape clicks off, I realize with great distress that Miranda has not come through in the reading. In fact, nobody has. I expected my entire session to be one big family reunion with departed relatives. He asks if I have any questions. I tell him I was hoping to hear from deceased loved ones—I had decided not to specifically mention a baby this time. He closes his eyes again and sits silently for a moment.

"There's a father figure here. Does the month of October mean anything to you?" he asks.

"Well, my grandpa passed away, but he died in the month of April."

"There's someone here named Mary. She wants you to tell her sister Rose that she's alright. Are those names familiar to you?"

"No, I don't think so," I answer, trying hard to remember the family tree.

Suddenly it comes to me. Al's cousin Mary Ellen died recently. She was young, in her forties I think. I know her sister as Rosemary, but she must have called her Rose.

Despite my disappointment, I cannot deny his ability. When he opens his eyes and tells me that is all, I leave the room feeling crushed. I still have no answers about Miranda. Later, when my mom and I compare notes, she tells me during her session her grandmother appeared to Edward holding a baby, although we can't be sure the baby is Miranda. Mom also reminds me that although Grandpa died in April, his birthday was in October.

~ ~ ~

This month's support group topic: Mother's Day one week ago. Many spent the morning or afternoon at a cemetery. Some of us received cards from friends and family. I am acutely aware that Beth, Heidi, Wendy, and I are fortunate to have a living child to dull the pain and give us something to celebrate. But for Dawn, Tracy, and Darlene, Mother's Day is a bitter reminder of what their lives could have been, should have been. I've learned that even though a woman becomes a mother from the moment of conception and will forever after remain a mother to that child regardless of his or her lifespan, many women question whether they can call themselves mother, especially when others fail to acknowledge them in that role.

"Andy went to a family party and couldn't understand why I was so upset and wouldn't go with him," Dawn tells us. "I told him I couldn't go and watch them be happy and not acknowledge me. I was so angry, I went to a bowling alley and hurled the ball at the pins, imagining they were Andy and his family. I had a very good game!" The room breaks into hysterical laughter. "Then one of Andy's relatives noticed my absence and said, 'What's her problem? She's not a mother anyway.' Andy came home as angry as me. No living children? Sorry, but your motherhood is being revoked. You no longer qualify!" smirks Dawn.

Tracy tells us about the April baptism of her goddaughter, Hannah, born a few months earlier. At first Tracy was bitter and angry. *Great, I get to be a godmother, but I can't have my own baby. This is my godchild by default because I can't have my own children,* thought Tracy during the baptism. Not used to feeling sorry for herself, she hated the emotions that were surfacing. But lately, her attitude has begun to change. "It's still hard, there are still tears and a little bitterness, and despite the painful reminder of what I'm missing with Paul, Hannah is growing on me," she says.

Wendy is still tormenting herself with thoughts of guilt and blame for David's death at sixteen weeks. "I'm a nurse. Why didn't I recognize the signs the night before my bag broke? Maybe this would have been different. Why didn't I know it was preterm labor? Maybe they could have given me medication." Adding to her guilt is the feeling she got pregnant too soon with David because she was trying to fix what was broken after her first miscarriage. She can't accept the idea that her fate is to keep losing babies. Wendy's depression has continued to worsen, prompting her counselor to write an advisory recommending Wendy take a leave of absence from work during the summer.

We talk for a few minutes after the meeting, and then Beth invites Wendy to join us at Omega. It had been a couple months since anyone new had joined us, and Beth's action saves her from my accusation of slacking off from her unspoken duties as club membership director.

~ ~ ~

At Omega, the conversation somehow leads to taxes.

"And then my accountant called and asked about a social security number for Madeline," continues Beth. "I told him I even have one for the dead one, Joshua, but that he only lived for two hours. He said it doesn't matter if he lived for two minutes, I still get the tax deduction. Can you believe that?"

"Hey, nobody told me I should get a tax deduction for Nathan," says Darlene.

"Yeah," says Dawn, "we applied for social security cards as soon as the triplets were born, and even though none of them made it, we were able to claim all of them on our tax return."

"That's not fair," I say. "I was pregnant four months longer than you, Beth, but Miranda didn't get a birth certificate, a social security number, or a tax deduction!"

"Tell everyone about your new job," says Heidi grinning at Darlene.

"I'm working at the Baby Superstore," Darlene tells us.

"What about the daycare center job you just started a few months ago?" I ask.

"I hated it," she says. "The owner's mother-in-law was so mean to some of the babies, I called DCFS on her."

"So, now instead of taking care of other people's babies, you're selling them things they need for their babies," I laugh.

"Yep," she says.

I look over at Wendy. "See what you've gotten yourself into? None of us are normal anymore."

~ ~ ~

"Wendy, where do you live?" I ask her on our way out to the parking lot.

"In the northwest suburbs."

"How long does it take you to drive here?"

"About forty-five minutes."

"That's a long way to drive home alone late at night."

"Oh, I don't mind."

As we all hug and say goodbye, I lean in to Wendy. "I'm really glad you came with us tonight," I whisper.

"Me too."

~ ~ ~

Driving home, I can't help but think about Wendy's story. While she shared more details with us tonight, I came to truly realize that the number of weeks her babies lived inside her—Kelly, thirteen weeks, and David, sixteen weeks—isn't the determining factor in the depth of her grief. I had already begun to suspect this during support group meetings, but Wendy is the first one I've met whose losses have all been before twenty weeks. Her baby's miscarriages have as much meaning for her as our losses have for us. Her pain is the same. No more. No less. No different.

22

Wendy's first pregnancy in 1993 had been a complicated one: at twenty-six weeks she had gone into premature labor, and although sent home with a medication pump to stop contractions, she ended up in the hospital every three weeks. Being a nurse, working both Labor and Delivery, as well as Critical Care Nursery, Wendy knew all the things that could go wrong. At thirty-seven weeks, the doctors turned the pump off, Wendy went into labor and Michael was born two days later, healthy as can be.

When Wendy found herself pregnant again, she was cautious. She knew she could experience more difficulties but remained hopeful and somewhat naïve. *This time could be different. Each pregnancy is different,* she told herself. At work she had access to an ultrasound machine, but she wasn't fanatical about it like another pregnant nurse on the floor who was constantly checking on her developing baby.

Wendy was doing a twelve-hour shift in the nursery. It was 5:30 p.m., quiet on the floor, and she asked a resident if he would do a quick ultrasound to check the baby's heartbeat. She was thirteen weeks into the pregnancy, almost past the critical first trimester, and had already heard the heartbeat at her first prenatal checkup. She went to Labor and Delivery happy and unworried. Three of her nurse friends stood by her side as they watched in anticipation for the small sac containing Wendy's quickly growing baby. The bedside ultrasound showed no sign of a heartbeat. They listened with the Doppler, but heard nothing. She remained unworried. The machines were simple bedside scanners, far from high-tech. *The baby is small. It's too early,* she told herself. Wendy shook it off and went back to work. The resident poked his head in the nursery where Wendy had returned and told her to go down to radiology where he had just scheduled a higher-level ultrasound. Maura, one of her friends, went down with her. It didn't occur to Wendy that anything could be wrong.

Sandy, the technician, searched for a visual of the heartbeat while Wendy relaxed on the exam table. She saw nothing with the abdominal probe and switched to the intravaginal ultrasound. Maura stood at the bedside next to Wendy while Sandy worked away, pushing buttons, neither woman speaking. "Well did you see the heartbeat?" Wendy finally asked.

"I can't say anything," answered Sandy.

"You're joking me!" she said.

Sandy hesitated.

"No, Wendy, there's no heartbeat," Sandy said.

Wendy's eyes flew open wide as if someone had stabbed her, and she burst into tears. "This can't happen to me. This can't happen to me. This can't happen to me," she cried. "My baby!"

Her OB came in and showed her the ultrasound pictures. The baby had developed for ten weeks and then stopped.

Wendy had the choice to wait for the baby to miscarry or schedule a dilation and curettage (D & C), a surgical procedure that would remove the fetal tissue from her uterus. The knowledge that she was carrying a dead baby was too horrible for her, and she called her husband, Mark, to come to the hospital and be with her during the D & C. That night, she pulled out a journal and began to write. She needed to keep track of her feelings, fearing she would forget, and so began an intimate relationship with an empty journal and a pen:

August 24, 1995

They told me you had no heartbeat. I cried as if someone had torn my heart from my chest, as if someone had taken every last space of air from my lungs, and as if every nerve was swelled with pain. How can you have no heartbeat? I only heard it for the first time nine days ago. The joyous, wondrous sound of life—gone. How can this happen to me, to us, little one? And why? Please, please dear Lord, let this be a nightmare. Please don't take my baby from me. I love her/him so much already. Remember, Lord, the day I heard this baby's heartbeat? Tears swelled in my eyes and I rejoiced in your goodness. Do I deserve this pain? Am I unfit? I pray for understanding. Hear me Lord. Do not let me drown in bitterness. Be with me. I need you so much.

I used to go to bed contented, full of life, full of you.

Now I go to bed empty, missing you.

I used to go to bed wondering how many times I would need to go to the bathroom.

Now I go to bed wondering how many times I will wake from my nightmare, pacing the floor, wandering from room to room, searching for a place to be, for a place to grieve.

I used to go to bed thinking, "only a few more nights of sleeping on my stomach."

Now I lay purposefully on my stomach missing you, yearning to have to turn on my side.

I used to go to bed listing in my head all the names we might call you.

Now I go to bed just calling you.

Every night, every day, every minute, every breath, you were with me.

Now you're gone.

Someone help me understand.

Wendy was devastated and couldn't believe her pregnancy was over. Her husband didn't get it and went back to work, leaving Wendy alone with Michael. Her mom, having given birth to six children and never experiencing a loss, couldn't relate to Wendy's grief and expected her to be over it after the first week. Wendy's youngest sister, Lisa, had no clue and hardly acknowledged Wendy's loss. Wendy's family, by nature, had always avoided difficult issues; they didn't talk about it, they ran from it. Adding to Wendy's grief was the fact that both her sister Lisa and her brother's wife, Donna, were also pregnant with their first babies. Wendy tried to be a good Christian, but her feelings of jealousy bordered on anger as the world passed her by. Isolated and depressed, she wasn't participating in life, but merely existing. Her sister Kelly, a psychologist and social worker, and her only source of support from the family, lived two hours away.

> *August 30, 1995*
>   *You've been gone a week. I think of you every morn-*
> *ing as I wake up and my belly is flat. I think of you as women*
> *with swelled abdomens pass by. I feel so alone. I will never be*
> *able to feel you move inside me. I won't ever touch your face,*
> *your baby skin. There were so many things I looked forward*
> *to, so many things like showing you to Michael for the first*
> *time, dressing you, bathing you, holding you, smelling you,*
> *putting you in a car seat next to your big brother Michael,*
> *watching you grow. Why did you die? I miss you so much.*
>   *She called you a miscarriage. I called you my baby.*
> *She said, "It's something that just happens"*
> *I think, "Why to you and me?"*
> *When did your heart stop beating?*
> *Were you in pain?*
> *Did you know I was falling in love with you?*
> *I'm sorry they had to take you from me that way.*
> *So sorry.*

> *A piece of my heart went with you.*
> *The tears keep falling.*
> *Are you with Him?*

September 2, 1995

I feel guilty for being on vacation. I'm starting to stuff the pain because I'm not supposed to grieve while I'm on vacation. We're in Ireland, where Mark is from. Drinking a lot because that's what they do here. I don't care what happens to me today. Isn't that terrible? It's Michael's birthday. Remembering his birth is joyful. Thanking the Lord for such a beautiful child, at the same time missing, grieving for the baby we lost. How can I keep going? No one here knows what's happening inside me.

September 6, 1995

We got home from Ireland tonight. I'm afraid of what lies ahead. The tears were perhaps prematurely interrupted. Will the flood gates open? I don't know how to think anymore. I'm different. Life is different. My baby is gone. My baby is gone. I want to cry. I don't.

September 7, 1995

I called Dr. Peterson's office to reschedule my appointment. I had to tell Lori I lost my baby and that I wanted to talk to Dr. Peterson instead of coming in for my monthly check-up. It hurts. How many women will come in to the office and take for granted the routine of the check-up? How many will take for granted their baby's heartbeat? I won't hear my little one's heartbeat tomorrow. I only heard it once. I only heard it once.

September 8, 1995

    I cried for you today. I miss you so much. Can anyone understand how much of my life was already invested in you? I'm lost without you. I don't know how to feel about my body. Someone I know saw me in the grocery store and asked how I was. I told her we lost you. She said she thought something was wrong because I "looked too thin." Where is my fat body with you growing inside? I was just getting used to my body changing and then you died. Why did this happen, little one?

September 10, 1995

    I worked yesterday for the first time since I lost you, little one. Many people, good people, offered their sympathies. I thank the Lord for their caring. Where would we be without human caring? How is it, then, that I still feel alone and lost? Could I ever even imagine it would be like this? I miss you.

    I took care of the babies in the nursery, lovingly, and in the midst of changing a diaper, holding a bottle to tiny lips, and wiping a mouth, I thought of you. I will never be able to take care of you this way. You are gone from me. I must think of you as being taken care of by the Lord. But are you? Because you were never born, does that mean you have no place with our God? Seems absurd. You were life. Life He created. I pray you have a very special place in heaven.

    Your big brother has helped me through this daily, nagging pain. You would have loved him. Right now he is discovering hiding his hands in his shirt sleeves and uncovering them. It has been wonderful watching him develop. I am so sad that I will miss that with you.

Although Wendy had been pregnant for only a few months, she had already connected with the life growing inside, planning and hoping for the future of her new child. She often thought about her two children being close in age and how they would play together. She remembered back to her own childhood when she and her sister did everything together. Her sister, although two years younger, was the same height, and they were often mistaken as twins. She wanted so much for Michael to have that special relationship with a sibling, to have someone next to him, to share things that he couldn't share with his parents.

September 14, 1995

> *I miss you. I talked to your Aunt Lisa today. She's going to have a baby around the time you were due. How am I going to make it through this? Every night I dream about you. I plead to the Lord for Him to give you back to me. Of course, every morning I wake and am reminded that you died.*

September 22, 1995
Dear Wendy,
To my beautiful daughter and my lost grandchild,

> *After reading your journal (I hope you don't care that I read it), I feel I let you down, but honey I do grieve for your lost little one. But I know in my heart that your little child is with God in heaven. I can't write the beautiful words that you can Wendy, but with tears streaming down my face as I write this, I feel your pain very much. I should have been with you that night. There are never the right words to say to someone who has lost something as precious as a child. I want to be there for you because you are my precious child, and when you hurt, I hurt. I know it will take time to get over this pain, but it will pass. When your little sister has her baby, you will be happy for her because you love her and her child and you are a very loving sister and aunt that wants the best for her as she*

*wants for you. Her happiness will also be yours because you
love life and God. Trust in Him!*
Love, Mom

September 29, 1995
     *Days have gone by since I've written. I think of you
everyday. Nights are still restless, full of dreams, most times of
babies. I guess you are still very much a part of me. I don't
want to ever forget you or your place in our family. You were
our second child. I think you need a name. Your dad and your
aunt say it's okay to call you Kelly. I hope it's alright to name
you this – we weren't able to determine if you were a boy or
a girl. I named you after my sister, your aunt. She's a good
and beautiful person. She's patient, genuine, persevering, kind,
loving – all the right qualities to have in this life. Our tiny
little angel Kelly. I feel comforted by this. I love you.*

October 8, 1995
     *I saw your pregnant Aunt Lisa today. I miss you
every day, yet today I longed for you. It's strange, little Kelly.
I think the sharp pain has passed, and then I see someone or
something and am reminded of you and your short little life.
You would be eighteen weeks by now. Incredible. Will I always
think this way?*
     *I am blessed to know the love of the Lord. I think of
you with Him and pray I will meet you someday. I miss you.
I still feel empty.*

October 12, 1995
     *It's a glorious day today. Indian summer, I would
imagine. Michael and I are at the park by the fire station.
Time to sit and think. Mark and I have been trying to conceive. Mark, passively—me, consciously. Truly I want a baby.*

Mark seems to take so many things for granted. He says we should "let it happen naturally." I, on the other hand, participate with my cycle. Am I too calculating or trying too hard? Maybe. I wish he could know what it means to harbor life, hold it precious, and then let it go.

Wendy felt selfish for wanting to move along so quickly; Mark wasn't ready, and although she didn't know if he even grieved over Kelly's loss, she felt he probably was more scared than she was.

December 1, 1995
Dear Kelly,

I'm going to have a baby! I'm overjoyed at the goodness of God in the conception of this baby, however I still miss you and think of you. I haven't written because I didn't want to feel sad. I am surprised by my feelings of still mourning you. Last weekend, Thanksgiving, someone asked your Aunt Donna when she was due. "March 7th," she replied, and her words stung like a bee—you were due then also—yet it wasn't like a knife going through me as it had been in the past.

Little tiny one, you will always be my second child in my heart. I love you. I am blessed.
Your mom

It was now February, sixteen weeks into her pregnancy, and Wendy had traveled two hours to her hometown for Donna's baby shower. The women were in the kitchen cutting up food for her mom's famous potato salad, when suddenly Wendy felt pressure down between her legs. She thought she had simply been standing too long, and her mom told her to sit down and relax. That night as she dreamt, a strong contraction jolted her awake. She got out of bed and called one of the residents at the hospital where she worked. He told her it could be one of two things: either she was going into premature labor, or she was dehydrated. He told her to drink some water and call him back in an hour. She went into the bathroom and suddenly felt pressure. She panicked, thinking the baby's head was coming out, and when she reached down to touch it she realized it was the amniotic sac. Suddenly the bag burst and fluid gushed out. Wendy screamed. Her mom, who came running in, didn't realize the implications of what had just happened, but Wendy knew.

At the hospital, everyone stood around telling her it was going to be okay as they did test after test to determine if her bag had actually broken. She was completely distraught insisting that it wasn't going to be okay. An ultrasound showed that the baby looked fine with a strong heartbeat and measurements that were on target for its gestational age.

They put Wendy in an ambulance and sent her to the hospital in Chicago where she worked. She rode alone for the ninety minute drive, the ambulance drivers quiet. When she got to the hospital, though staff knew her, they talked around her, not to her.

Mark, who had been home taking care of Michael, met her there, and her OB came in to discuss their options. Her cervix wasn't yet dilated, but there wasn't much they could do for a sixteen-week gestation baby if she delivered now. There were isolated cases of babies being kept alive in utero until twenty-four weeks, but the risks of infection to the baby and to Wendy were serious. If infection developed in her uterus and went untreated, she would risk losing not only the baby, but her uterus and with it the possibility of ever having another baby again. "I'm not that courageous," she told him. "I want to have more children." Wendy could also choose to induce labor, but it would mean almost a certain death sentence for her baby. How could she make such a choice? Wendy hoped the doctors would make the decision for her.

That night, as Mark slept on a mattress on the floor, Wendy lay awake alone with her thoughts and turned to her journal.

February 17, 1996

Sometimes we all wish we had the power to change the past. Today was one of those times. Somehow I think if I paid attention to the cramping, this little baby would have had a chance. I would give anything to change what lies ahead of us. I feel as though I've left the baby unprotected, to come into this world without a chance to breathe, to cry, to touch, to know.

So here I am again with pen in hand in an emotional hell, trying to come to terms with the inevitable death of another baby. I can't believe I have to let another baby go— go home to where he or she belongs. I pray that in heaven this baby will breathe, will touch, will sing beside the Lord. I pray this baby will know how much he/she was wanted and loved.

"Lord, please take this cup from me not as I would have it, but according to your will." Remember those words? I understand them more than I would dare admit. Please, Lord, help me through this. Don't let my baby suffer. Be here. I feel so weak. Help me understand your love in the midst of this insufferable pain. Hold me. Hold Mark.

Dear baby of mine,

Where can I begin to tell you of our hopes and dreams for you? I must tell you I was hesitant in thinking about you and your future because of Kelly, the baby that died before you. However, I did begin to dream about you and looked forward to harboring you for many more weeks. Just a couple of days ago, your father and I talked about names. We will name you because you were a part of us and you deserve at least a name.

This morning, as we looked at you through ultrasound and as your heart beat about 140, I thanked God that I could at least see your image and know you were alive.

I secretly cried, asking your forgiveness for being an incompe-
tent vessel. You are my baby. I can't let you go.
Love,
Mom

As usual, Labor and Delivery was full—it was always a zoo—
and a resident came in and told the nurses to move Wendy to the postpartum floor and let her deliver the baby there. The postpartum nurses
wouldn't be too happy about it; they took care of moms and babies
and weren't used to dealing with premature infants, many of whom
died in their mother's arms. Wendy knew she would hear babies crying all night or see them breastfeeding out in the hall and wanted to
stay in Labor and Delivery.

"Too bad," the nurses told the resident, "we're not moving
her," and they convinced Wendy's OB to write orders keeping Wendy
in Labor and Delivery. She found some solace in the fact that the
nurses caring for her were her friends, good friends, but yet they were
walking on eggshells, afraid to say anything to her. They weren't ver-
balizing their feelings and compassion, and any communication or
comforting had to be initiated by Wendy. *My baby is dying, my whole
entire being is going away from me,* she needed them to understand.

This time, Mark understood, breaking down in the cafeteria
while Wendy's dad sat helpless, unable to do anything for his daughter
and son-in-law.

February 19, 1996
    Fr. Martin visited me today. The Lord was with me.
We talked about life sustaining measures and, in our belief,
the Lord does not require us to go beyond extraordinary
means. Fr. Martin spoke of the rupture of membranes as the
deciding factor in my baby's fate. He drew similarities in the
baby to a terminally ill patient. We know that they will die,
it's a matter of when to withdraw the life support. He made

so much sense. He took the burden of the thinking that I would be the cause of the baby's death from my shoulders. I felt stronger. I had to move on.

We checked the baby's heart rate at 5:30 p.m. – 180s. Dear Lord, is he suffering? My temperature is going up. At 7 p.m. we started the induction. How will I ever get through this?

They gave Wendy medication to alleviate pain and help her relax, but it made her foggy. They wouldn't give her an epidural, yet the pain was just as intense as when she had delivered Michael, and for four hours she felt like she was being torn apart.

The baby was alive up until his delivery, but when he finally emerged, his heart had stopped beating. Wendy cried until she had no tears left. Even though she had no control over her bag breaking, she felt in the end she had pulled the plug on her son and couldn't bear the thought that she caused her baby's death by pushing him into the world.

A nurse wrapped him in a blue towel and put him in a placenta basin. Wendy looked at him while they took Polaroid photos, but she didn't hold him and nobody offered or asked her if she wanted to. Mark didn't look at the baby, whom they named David.

February 19, 1996

David was born at 9:30 p.m. So, so very little, yet perfect. Maura and Linda baptized him. During labor, his heart had stopped beating sometime along the way. I looked at him and wondered, Would he have been a round, fat thing? Would he have given Michael a run for his money? They would have been great buddies. What is Mark feeling in all of this? I looked at David yet couldn't cry. So many tears before this moment. I just feel as though I've failed him in some way. Lord help me. Help me.

My dear sweet baby,
*   You looked perfect. Only time would help you grow.*
Why was time taken away from you? Why did your life have
to end? My dear sweet tiny David, even too little to hold
close. Why didn't I take you from that tray and hold you near
my heart? How will I make it through the night? I am lost.
Nothing matters. I am empty. You are gone from me.

Wendy was moved to a quiet room on the postpartum floor
the next morning and had to stay all day and night for antibiotic treatment. Mark went back to work while her sister, Kelly, took care of
Michael. Wendy's parents went back home and Wendy was left in the
hospital to grieve alone.

Wendy was confronted with the question of what to do with
David's body. Both considered miscarriages, David had only been three
weeks older than Kelly, yet Kelly had been removed via D & C, a medical procedure, and David had been delivered and photographed. If she
chose not to make any arrangements, the baby would be buried in a
common grave.

February 20, 1996
*   People stopping by my room to inquire about my*
welfare. Oddly, I want them near to validate the death of my
baby. However, I want them to go away because my pain is so
great. Marianne, Sharon, Maura, Amy, Lila, Teresa, Paula—
all there. Thank you Lord for such caring people in my life. I
feel ungrateful, numb, empty. Guilt for even feeling.
*   Sister Mary helped me plan David's funeral and*
burial. Thank you Lord. She is a gift. She is your presence.
Mark and I will bury him as he was so much a part of our
lives for sixteen weeks.
*   Tears keep falling, tears keep falling.*

Mark came back Wednesday to take Wendy home. The funeral home put David in a little white box and took him to a small $75 lot in the children's section of the cemetery for a graveside funeral service. Sister Nancy, from Wendy's church, performed the service, telling a story about the mystery of life and death and our limited understanding. She concluded with prayer and they went home.

On the day they buried David, Wendy's sister-in-law Donna gave birth to a son. It had been his baby shower that Wendy had been preparing for when her water bag broke. Wendy's mom and dad, who had been with her and Mark at the cemetery, left quickly to be with Wendy's brother and his wife for the delivery. Wendy's sister Lisa had already given birth to a healthy baby girl the month before David's death; now there were two newborns in the family. Wendy was devastated and felt rejected and abandoned.

> *February 27, 1996*
> *I understand that I had David for what might seem a mere moment as compared with lifelong spouses, siblings, mothers, fathers or even children. But David was my baby whom I looked forward to rearing and loving. The red hotness manifests itself in being cheated of a memory.*
> *I dread tonight.*
> *Lord, you are my life. David is with the Lord, rejoined to Him whole.*

It was February, cold and dark, and Wendy quickly slipped into depression. She wondered what was wrong with her that nobody was coming to her side to give her support, to hold her together. She expected more connection with Mark after David's death. What she didn't expect were the feelings of isolation that plagued her every moment. The baby was formed, it was more real, this was Mark's second son. And yet, Mark's reaction was the same as it had been after the loss of baby Kelly: go to work and don't talk about it. Wendy found it easier to talk about David with two-and-a-half-year-old Michael than with Mark. "Why?" he asked, when she told him the baby had died. She told him that the baby's bubble of water had popped and he couldn't live without it. "Well, why did it pop?" he asked.

"I wish I could tell you," she answered.

She took Michael to the cemetery to see where his baby brother was now. The children's section was adorned with toys and windmills, and it was like a playground to Michael. Wendy's parents bought a stone engraved with David's name and the words *Safe in the Arms of Jesus, February 19th, 1996.* It had a picture of a little boy holding a lamb. Perhaps the only comfort she found was that if she couldn't hold him then the Lord was holding him.

Wendy went back to her part-time job in the nursery after three weeks, but soon began having difficulty doing her job. Suddenly the babies she was caring for in the nursery were much more fragile to her. Before she was able to look at her charges as patients, but now they were "somebody's baby." She couldn't stand to hurt the babies, and if she didn't get an IV into an infant on the first try, she would stop. Her confidence in her nursing skills dwindled.

Babies born too premature to survive were often brought up to the nursery for comfort measures such as a warming bed and photos. When she would come into work and see a premature baby listed on the board she would refuse to take it. Nobody gave her a hard time about it, but after a while she worried that she was burdening her coworkers and felt bad about herself.

She no longer felt connected to her friends at work and didn't talk to them on the same level she had before. They had disappointed her. During her delivery they had followed the checklist of what to do when a baby was born early or dead, and they stopped by to check on her, but did nothing more. *It was just ignorance on their part,* she rationalized, but couldn't help but feel angry.

One of Wendy's nurse friends told her about a woman named Pat Vaci she had met at a support group after suffering her own miscarriage. Wendy talked with Pat several times after David's death, and Pat encouraged Wendy to come to the support group meetings, but also put Wendy in touch with a counselor, an older woman who had experience with mothers and grief after a loss. In March, Mark, who was resistant to Wendy seeking therapy, took her to her first counseling appointment. "I could have told you all the things she just told you," he said after the first session. But Wendy didn't think she could survive without this woman and would continue the relationship for three years.

It was spring and the cold weather was finally letting up. Wendy felt lost and alone and needed to get out, but she couldn't bear to take Michael to the park because there always seemed to be a pregnant woman, and Wendy's head would be flooded with thoughts of jealousy and meanness. So she stayed in the house feeling increasingly isolated.

~ ~ ~

Mark's dad died in April and they traveled to Ireland for the funeral. There were a few tears, a few drinks, lots of stories, and the next day they were all back to work.

Mark had now lost two babies and a father within one year, but he held it all in. Mark's family offered some support to Wendy only after checking with Mark to see how Wendy was doing and whether it was safe to bring up the subject of David. But they were consumed with grief for Mark's father, and Wendy was still so consumed by her own grief she felt completely removed from her father-in-law's funeral.

April 11, 1996
    I haven't written in a long time. I can't. I have no words. I... am I nothing?

23

It's June 20th, 1996, the first anniversary of Miranda's death. Or, is it her birthday? I don't know what to call it. Regardless of what it is, I'm dreading it. It's not that I miss her more today. It's just that the feelings seem to be bubbling up like lava from a previously dormant volcano.

So here I am in my new house—a house with cabinet locks left behind by the previous owners that I don't need because I don't have a one-year-old to keep out of the cabinets—wondering if I should be sitting in quiet solitude or throwing a birthday party. I know I can't treat this like any other day. Miranda deserves something. I need something.

I realize that today and on each anniversary for the rest of my life, I'll wonder what she would be doing now. This year, her first year, she would be playing peek-a-boo and pat-a-cake, taking her first wobbly steps, smiling at us with birthday cake smashed all over her face, calling out to Mama and Dada, and giving us sweet baby kisses.

I would be pushing around the big double stroller, Alex turning around to make faces at her giggling baby sister; portrait studio photos with matching outfits, Alex's arms wrapped around Miranda to keep her from falling over or scooting away; going to a restaurant and asking for a booster seat *and* a high chair. And that's only the first year.

What about potty training and preschool? The first day of kindergarten and the first loose tooth? Baking cookies and making mud pies and reading *Go Dog Go,* my favorite childhood book by Dr. Seuss? And on and on… My dreams for this child filled a lifetime.

My closest family and friends have remembered with calls or cards, which means more to me than they could possibly know. Rachel's note says that she thinks of Miranda every day when she's thinking of Sean. Although Al's mom hasn't verbally acknowledged Miranda today, I saw "Miranda's Birthday" written on her calendar. She remembers.

As I contemplate today, I sit on the couch staring up at the angel plate on the mantel, hoping for inspiration. Other than Miranda's photo, which sits on my bedroom dresser, this is the only other visible reminder of her in my house, and I smile remembering the events that led up to the arrival of my angel plate.

It was late last summer when I began looking for the perfect substitute for Miranda's photo, which I couldn't yet bring myself to put up on the mantel. During the next five months, mail-order angel dolls came and went—I couldn't find the perfect thing—until I came across an offer in the mail one day for an angel painted on a collector's plate that made my mouth drop open. This might have been what my baby would have looked like had she lived. The similarities between the angel and Miranda were eerie. Both had dark hair and pink cheeks, long eyelashes, and heads cocked slightly to one side. Both wore gowns of pink and white, and while Miranda's gown had white bunnies on it with a pink ribbon, at the feet of the angel sat a white bunny draped in a pink ribbon.

But I hesitated; I'd been disappointed so many times already. A few days later, the same picture was blowing by me on the ground as I took my daily walk. Surely, it was a sign. I ordered one for myself and my mom, hurt that Al's mom had declined the offer, until the day I walked into her bedroom and was stopped in my tracks by the sight of Miranda's photo on her dresser in a frame that said *My Guardian Angel,* my heart swelling with love and appreciation for my mother-in-law.

My angel plate, although beautiful, is a poor substitute for a child, and my heart sinks at the prospect of trying to plan a day that will honor and remember her without an emotional tidal wave washing me out to sea. The phone rings; it's my mom, come to the rescue, inviting Alex and me down to Indiana for a day at the beach.

Stretched out on the hot sand, I pull out a notebook from my bag and let my feelings flow out.

As I sit on the shore of Lake Michigan, a place I came often as a child, watching Alex play in the sand and romp in the waves, I reflect on the past year.

I've been to hell and back. I want to believe I will never again suffer so much pain. But I must accept the reality that there are no guarantees.

Everyone told me the first year would be the hardest, and I told myself that if I could just get through the first year everything would be okay. I did, and it was. I can smile again, laugh again, enjoy the things I once loved. But I am a changed person. No longer can I learn of tragedy without being affected and reminded. No longer can I take pregnancy and childbirth for granted. No longer do I naively expect to live a long life, growing old with my husband, watching our children have children. I hope, but do not expect. Life's smaller disappointments no longer have a hold on me; they simply don't matter from a soul's perspective.

I have grown: as a wife, mother, human being. I wouldn't have become this person without the gift of Miranda's life. I wonder what she has gained by coming to us for her brief moment. I know someday I'll have that answer— she'll tell me in her own words as we walk, hand in hand, perhaps along a shore not so different from this one.

My attention is drawn to Alex as she drags my mom by the hand down to the water's edge to show her some treasure, perhaps a shell or a shiny rock, and I smile, thinking that as a young child I must have done the same to my mother.

When we get home that night, we stick a candle into a cupcake and sing "Happy Birthday" to Miranda. Alex blows out the candle as I watch Al, wondering what he's thinking. In the background, a single white candle silently burns on the mantel in remembrance.

~ ~ ~

The June support group meeting will be my last. I feel like I've come full circle with grieving. I hadn't realized it until one recent day when I asked my brother-in-law for Miranda's ashes. The day he brought them, I had no idea what to expect; I had never seen the cremated remains of anyone. He handed me a small, white cardboard box labeled with Miranda's name and cremation date; crude for the remains of a baby, yet I liked the simplicity. I lifted open the flap and found white tissue paper, as if I was opening a gift. The white plastic bag underneath was just small enough to fit neatly in the palm of my hand and just thin enough to see the small chips of black, gray, and white rock-like substance inside. I chuckled at the irony of the final resting place of Miranda's cremated remains—a fireproof safe.

It's been one year and although I realize I will never get over losing Miranda, I've slowly been embracing life again and feel ready to put grief behind me. Many of the people I've journeyed with over the past year are expecting subsequent babies and have already stopped coming. Dawn, although not pregnant, doesn't feel a strong need to be here, and her attendance has become sporadic. As I walk down the hall to our meeting room, I tell myself that the next time I walk through the doors of this hospital, I intend it to be with a bulging belly, ready to give birth.

We're talking about signs from our babies, or feeling our babies' presence around us. My friend Sher told me that if I asked Miranda to give me a sign, although I might have to ask several times, she would let me know she was still with me. In the beginning, I was almost too afraid to ask. Not because I feared she would answer, but because I feared she would not. Or that if she did answer, I might miss it or misinterpret it. And where would that leave me? Although I had a strong belief in the afterlife, or the other side, I wasn't sure if Miranda had access to my feelings, my thoughts, my love, or whether she could return those intangible things to me.

A woman named Kristi, who has lost triplets, tells us she came home one day and found three baby bunnies sitting in her backyard. She immediately called her husband at work. As Kristi stood on the deck in amazement, the bunnies ran circles around the tree in the center of their backyard. They seemed happy and playful. "I wish you were here to see this," Kristi told her husband. Later that same day, in the early evening, when Kristi's husband arrived home from work, the bunnies were there to greet him, and once again played in the yard while he watched in wonder.

I know if Dawn were here she would be sharing her stories of seeing the birds on her deck, always in groups of three.

Tracy shares that on one particularly sad day, she asked God to please give her a sign that Paul was with her. Suddenly a deer jumped out from a grove of trees, and Tracy's heart jumped as she smiled. She also admits that at home she often sees a flutter out of the corner of her eye, and although she can never quite make out a form, she has an undeniably strong feeling it's Paul.

Beth tells us one night three months after Josh died, in the deepest part of her depression, she sat in bed reading a book about angels, following the advice of her counselor who urged her to get in touch with Joshua's spirituality. Suddenly a scent filled the air around her, and although she had no flowers in her room, no perfume, nor anything else that could be producing such a smell, she was certain the scent was that of roses. She sniffed the book, her bedding, her nightgown, but the scent was gone. She looked back down at her book and read the very next sentence. "You may even smell the scent of an angel:

jasmine or rose." Beth began to sob. It was a turning point in her healing. Heidi says she has also smelled roses, in her car.

Darlene, while blasting her special song for the twins—Mariah Carey's "One Sweet Day," about a loved one who's flown away to heaven and waiting to meet again—heard knocking on her apartment door, five knocks three separate times. Each time she opened the door there was nobody there, yet the layout of the hall wouldn't allow for someone to knock and run without being seen. She closed the door, dropped to the floor and sobbed, knowing it was her boys telling her they were still with her.

My life isn't completely void of unexplainable events. I tell them about my double rainbow a few days after Miranda's death, which I too believe was the sign I had been pleading for. What I don't tell them about is the number sequences I've been seeing on clocks ever since Miranda left, always the same digits in a row: 111, 222, 333, sometimes every day for weeks at a time. Sometimes it happens more than once a day. Books I've read say this is angel communication. Spiritual friends tell me it's a message from a loved one. I don't know exactly what it means for me, but it always warms my heart and makes me smile, giving me a sense that I'm not alone. A musical toy has played twice by itself; I've heard whispers that sound like someone's calling "Mom" to me, yet when I search nearby rooms, nobody is around; and then there was the incident at the outdoor concert last summer.

It had only been a month since we'd lost Miranda. Al and I were lying on a blanket in the grass, on a beautiful summer night, with a light breeze and a gorgeous sunset, listening to the band and watching Alex dance. I was thinking I should be nursing an infant at my breast. And changing her diaper. And dancing with her in my arms. I was pulled from my longing by a white feathery, silky ball hovering around me—my naturalist friend, Jessica, would later identify it as a seedling from a Cottonwood tree—looking like the stuff angel wings must be made of. *A flying fluff,* I called it.

I reached up and watched it dance around my hand. It swirled up and down and around me, never straying too far, ignoring the breeze that begged to carry it away. My heart beat fast with excitement and wonder. It should have been long gone. *What's happening?* I asked the universe. *Is that you Miranda, telling me you're here?* Or was I losing my mind?

I looked away to watch Alex, expecting the flying fluff to be gone when my eyes returned, but it was still there, dancing playfully. Needing to know her spirit was with me, I had been praying for a sign from Miranda that she was alright. An unlikely means of communication, was this the answer I had been waiting for? After several minutes it finally drifted up and away, caught in the gentle breeze.

~ ~ ~

After the meeting, at Omega, Tracy announces with excitement she's pregnant again. She's already looking ahead to the February due date, time off work, day care plans, etc. Like Heidi who's struggling to prepare for her new baby while simultaneously grieving Brittany, emotionally Tracy is a wreck. Her doctor and staff have sensed her turmoil and do what they can to ease her anxiety and reassure her with weekly ultrasounds. Up until the discovery of her pregnancy, it was still hard for Tracy to look at pregnant women. Now her entire thinking about pregnancy has had to change. *Be confident, but tread lightly because you just don't know. You can't take anything for granted anymore,* she constantly tells herself.

Along with adjusting to a new pregnancy, she and Jim have decided to sell their "bachelor" house with no kitchen. "The nursery hasn't been touched for eight months. It must seem bizarre to prospective buyers. They don't see any sign of a baby. They can't tell I'm pregnant. They must think I'm weird," she says.

I'm thinking how wonderful this is for Tracy, praying all goes well for her this time. And yet, I'm beginning to feel that a new club is evolving—*The Good News Club*—and I wonder if I'll be a part of it or get left behind.

24

From my bedroom window I can see a slice of the horse farm across the street. Figures of ebony, white, and chestnut stand lazily grazing while the sun beats on their backs. Suddenly from behind a grove of trees bursts a young black stallion running and kicking in a playful charge. My view of this magnificent creature lasts only two seconds—a mere fraction of my day—before he disappears behind the trees again. But it's just long enough to take my breath away and leave me exhilarated at the mere thought of him, not unlike Miranda, who in a flash flew into my life, kicked in my womb, taking my breath away, and was suddenly gone—a mere fraction of my life.

Watching the horses is one of my favorite things to do in the summer, and the days have easily rolled into July, perhaps my favorite of all the months. Al and I look forward to a carefree summer and the start of a new emotional year. When my period doesn't come this month, I try to suppress my excitement; I've been disappointed so many times during the past year. I let myself buy a pregnancy test but then make myself put it away, not ready to face the disappointment of a negative result. Today, I would rather bask in the possibility.

Each day goes by, and the excitement grows. Finally, I can't stand it anymore and run upstairs to the bathroom. After peeing on the stick, I wait in the bedroom on the edge of the bed watching the clock while my heart pounds for five long minutes. When I walk back into the bathroom, I'm afraid to look at the stick. Holding my breath, I open my eyes, look down, and draw in a deep breath. There's a faint line! The shock is quickly replaced with an exhilaration I can hardly contain. "Oh my God, I'm pregnant. Oh my God!" I whisper to myself.

I know the day it happened. Al had come home from a three-day business trip on a hot, steamy day, and for the first time in a year, we made love for no reason other than sheer desire.

I race downstairs and find Al outside, sitting on the steps of the deck. Sitting down beside him, I hand him the test stick. "What's this?" he asks.

"What do you think it is?" I answer, giving him a shove.

He wraps his arms around me and holds me for a moment. Then he gives his typical response: "You'd better go see the doctor and make sure."

My family arrives soon after for a Fourth of July cookout and, too excited to keep the secret, I blurt out my announcement before they get to the front door.

Two days later, there's blood in the toilet. I've never bled during a pregnancy and begin to shake with nausea. *This can't be happening, not after all I've been through,* I tell myself. The feelings and thoughts from that night in June one year earlier come flooding back; it's like losing Miranda all over again. Sitting on the floor, my back braced against a wall, I nervously call my friend Lynne, knowing she bled during her pregnancies. She calms me down and tells me to call Dr. Ross, who coincidentally is also her OB. It's a Saturday and the office is closed; I know any one of the doctors might be on call right now, and my odds of getting Dr. Ross are slim. After the answering service asks all the routine questions—name, number, and complaint—I ask who's on call. "Dr. Ross," she says, and I breathe a sigh of relief. A few minutes later the phone rings and I hear his reassuring voice. He tells me it's perfectly normal for some women to bleed during pregnancy. He wants me to take it easy and call if the bleeding gets worse or I begin having painful cramps.

The next day, we drive to a country lake for a relaxing week by the pool and on the beach. The bleeding continues, but is sporadic and light. *Everything is going to be fine,* I tell myself over and over. But by Tuesday the trickle becomes a river and cramping has me clutching my abdomen in pain. When I pass a large clot in the bathroom, I slump to the floor and break down sobbing. "Oh God, no, my baby!"

I know I'm losing the pregnancy, and there's nothing I or anyone else can do to stop it. The nurse at Dr. Ross's office gently tells me over the phone to try to bring home any large pieces of tissue I can recover in case it needs to be examined. I drop my hand into the cold toilet water and scoop up the blood-soaked mass I assume is my undeveloped baby. Slipping it into a plastic bag, I hide it in the refrigerator. I try to keep up appearances for Al and Alex, but as the bleeding and cramping become unbearable, my world comes crashing down on me.

In my mind, that positive pregnancy test, the absence of menstruation, the early stages of nausea, represented a child in the making. Although I never heard or saw a heartbeat, conception had occurred, and I envisioned an embryo growing minute by minute into my much-wanted baby.

When we return home, I drive directly to Dr. Ross's office. When he walks by and sees me in the waiting room, once again he comes out, wraps his arms around me, and immediately takes me back to the ultrasound room to look for any sign of a developing embryo. For a few brief moments I have hope again.

As Dr. Ross preps me for the ultrasound, my mind drifts off to the day I met him, my first prenatal checkup when I was newly pregnant with Alex. While he searched for the heartbeat, he sang a silly song, endearing me to him instantly. The sound of a slow, steady beat floated through the room. "Is that the baby?" I'd asked with excitement. "No, that's you," he'd said, smiling. "Oh." Then suddenly another rhythm, this one faster, filled the air and I looked up at him. "That's your baby," he said. Tears filled my eyes, and he asked where my husband was. "Working," I'd answered. "Bring him with next time so he can hear this too," he'd said, and I'd nodded, unable to speak.

"Monica, there's nothing here," he says, the sound of his voice pulling me back to the present. Looking at the blank screen, my heart sinks. "Maybe you're wrong on your dates and it's too early to see the sac," he says. I know that isn't the case and have already given up on the pregnancy—a pregnancy ended in miscarriage at six weeks. "I'm sorry," he says. "Are you okay?" I nod my head and try to swallow the lump growing in my throat.

"I was expecting this," I tell him.

"At least you know you can get pregnant on your own," he says.

I can only nod again.

Now that all hope has been crushed and reality sets in, I feel the emotions building as I leave the office in search of Pat Vaci in the adjoining hospital building. A nurse on the maternity floor tells me she's in the Atrium eating lunch. When my eyes meet Pat's, I can no longer hold back the tears. She puts her arm around me, excuses herself from her lunch with a coworker and walks me out into the hall. We sit down on a bench, and she asks me to tell her everything. She's supportive and compassionate, and after pouring out two weeks worth of pent-up emotions, I take a deep breath and begin to feel better just as Dr. Ross walks up to us.

"I'm glad you found Pat," he smiles, laying his hand on my shoulder. "I was worried about you."

One week later, after the bleeding finally stops, I have to go in for a hormone check to make sure my body has rid itself of all the pregnancy tissue. In the second month of pregnancy, my hCG hormone level should have numbered well into the tens of thousands. The nurse calls the next day and tells me my level is three. Then she apologizes. *Three.* How ridiculous the number sounds, a slap in the face after all I've been through during the past year.

As I struggled to get pregnant for nearly one year, I gained a greater awareness and sensitivity to women's difficulty with infertility. Now I must add one more dimension of pregnancy loss to my experience: miscarriage. Now I understand a little more what Wendy and Dawn have gone through.

Dr. Ross told me I can try to get pregnant again as soon as I want. I call relatives and friends who've lost babies to miscarriage and learn several of them got pregnant again soon afterwards, which gives me hope.

The very next day, I'm back in Dr. Ross's office for a urinalysis. Diagnosis: urinary tract infection. Two weeks later, I'm back again for my annual physical and Pap smear. All I really want is a prenatal visit.

~ ~ ~

Later that month, at my ten-year high school class reunion, I walk over to the front corner of the room to look at the poster-size photos of our three classmates who have died, one during high school, the other two after graduation. Looking at the photo of Eric, who ran cross country with my brother Brian and was the first true love of my friend Jessica, I'm reminded of a conversation I had with a former friend who had called on behalf of the reunion committee just months earlier.

"You listed your stillborn baby on the questionnaire," she had said on the phone. They were printing a booklet to hand out at the reunion and asked us to send in our children's names and dates of birth. Only a few close friends knew about Miranda, but I had decided everyone should know, including the Morton High School class of 86. I wasn't sure why because it was unlikely I would ever see these people again. I wasn't looking for sympathy. I finally realized it was because I wanted to heighten public awareness about pregnancy and infant loss. I thought, also, that maybe someone who wasn't appreciating their own kids would go home and give them an extra hug. So I wrote down both of my children's names, adding that Miranda was stillborn, and sent it in.

"Yes, I did list my stillborn baby on the questionnaire," I answered her.

"Did you want us to print that in the booklet?" she asked with hesitation.

"Yes, I want you to print it," I told her, trying to remain calm. I wanted to ask her if she was planning on printing anything about Eric, our classmate who was killed on his bicycle by a hit-and-run driver, and when she said yes, I would ask her if she thought Eric was any more real to his mother as she cried over his dead body than Miranda was to me as I cried over hers, and why she would expect me to exclude one of my children, albeit a dead one. But she was a nice person, and I didn't have the heart to interrogate her. I thanked her for the call and quickly hung up.

As Eric's photo smiles at me, I smile back, remembering his laugh and wondering how his mother is now, ten years later.

Throughout the evening, as classmates talk about jobs and degrees, which I'm finding increasingly mundane, I keep my ears open for anyone who has had a pregnancy-related loss. It doesn't take long. My friend Jessica whispers to me that one of our mutual friends has had several miscarriages. I look over and watch my friend's face as everyone else shows off pictures of their kids, and I'm probably the only one who knows what she's thinking. I quickly pull her aside and tell her I know and how sorry I am, giving her a hug. She smiles, and we sit down and share about our losses, grateful to have found each other, even if only for one night.

~ ~ ~

It's August, hot and sweaty, and I'm determined to make a good effort towards conception. But Al is starting to come down with something and doesn't feel well. By the third night of premeditated, calculated sex, he is clearly irritated with me. I watch the calendar closely that month. Day 28 comes and goes. Then day 29, day 30, day 31.

My period is late.

Each day I become more hopeful but keep the secret suspicion to myself, waiting a full week until I can't stand it anymore and slip into the bathroom to take a pregnancy test. Once again my heart pounds for five minutes while I sit on the edge of the bed waiting. When I walk back in to check the results, I waste no time.

Positive.

I sigh with relief. This time the line is much darker than the last time, and I hope this is a good sign.

My emotions swirl around each other like oil and water: ecstatic to be pregnant again, yet fully expecting it to end. It takes several days to bring myself to tell Al he might be a father again, and my indifference is evident when I casually drop the news on him while standing in a checkout lane at the store. His response tells me he shares my guarded attitude.

I call only a few friends—Kathy, Lynne, and Beth, who tells the other five in our group—keeping the news even from my parents, afraid to get their hopes up again. If I tell anyone else, I'll be expected to act happy and excited. I don't feel that way and don't want to put on a "dog and pony show," as Heidi likes to say.

During the weeks that follow, my fear of losing the pregnancy grows with each passing day. Every time I go to the bathroom, I look down nervously expecting to see blood. At an out-of-town wedding reception, in the bathroom, I wipe and see blood. The hot nausea washes over me as that sinking feeling hits me once more. Why, why is this happening again? I'm shaking when I come out and Al knows something is wrong. When I tell him, he puts his arms around me and holds me tight.

I haven't been drinking alcohol, but what's the point of abstaining now? With a glass of wine to soothe my nerves, I keep a smile on my face pretending to have a good time, sinking into a sofa to avoid attention, crumbling on the inside.

The spotting clears up after a few days, and in October I go, with Alex in tow, for my first prenatal exam, supposedly eight weeks pregnant, already feeling the morning sickness. Lying on the ultrasound table, I keep my eyes off the screen and try to relax as Alex watches with curiosity from across the room. *What if something is wrong? What if there is no baby?* Dr. Ross points the vaginal scope in different directions while I wait.

"There," he says. I quickly turn toward the monitor. A small sac appears like a circle of light, enveloping the tiny life inside me, the flutter of a beating heart. I'm overcome with relief and a moment of joy as tears stream down my face. He takes my hand and gives it a gentle squeeze. I call Alex to come over and look. Hesitant, she obliges me, but the image fails to hold her attention and she quickly leaves my side to go back to her book. Dr. Ross says everything looks perfect and gives me a due date of May 20th.

I spend the next few months in a state of paranoia, afraid of miscarrying. My morning sickness is now around-the-clock, and when some friends ask me to come along on a weekend getaway, I reluctantly turn them down and spend the entire weekend sick on the couch.

The days drag as I count off gestational weeks on the calendar trying to get through the first trimester. I'll think about the rest of the pregnancy later if I even make it to thirteen weeks.

25

The cold winds of December are blowing as I mark off week sixteen on my calendar. Although I know it's too early and I shouldn't expect to feel movement from the baby, the lack of it keeps me on edge. It's difficult to go on every day wondering if my baby is alive or dead.

At my appointment, I'm surprised when Dr. Ross's nurse takes me into the ultrasound room again. I suspect Dr. Ross is sneaking me in here each month, unbeknownst to the scrutinizing eyes of the Gestapo manager in the front office, and I'm grateful for the special attention. Although he's never said so, I think he's as anxious as I am to get this baby safely into the world.

I watch the screen waiting for any sign of movement. Four weeks ago, after my twelve-week appointment confirmed I was still carrying a baby with a heartbeat, we put on our happy faces and told our family and friends about the baby, but our worry overshadowed any joy that we could muster. My "wait-and-see" attitude made it awkward to tell people our "big news." With six long months to get through, I wouldn't be able to breathe a sigh of relief until this baby was in my arms, alive.

When the visual of my baby comes on the screen, it's difficult to pinpoint the beating heart amidst the movement of tiny limbs. Dr. Ross points out the facial features, heart, arms and legs, hands and feet. Not only does life still live inside of me, it appears to be flourishing.

I ask Dr. Ross if there's any indication of the sex of the baby. I never wanted to know with Alex or Miranda, but now everything about pregnancy is different for me. As Heidi put it when she became pregnant again after Brittany, "Knowing that the baby was a girl was my way of getting to know her as much as I could right from the start in case she died, too." Dr. Ross says he doesn't see any signs of male anatomy, but it's still too early to tell for sure. It doesn't matter. I have a baby with a heartbeat; that's all I care about.

~ ~ ~

Since I've stopped going to support group meetings and have been too sick to meet anyone at Omega, I'm eager to see my six friends at the Christmas memorial service. For the first time, I've brought a special companion other than my husband. Alex, who's almost four now, is finally old enough to sit quietly, and understands enough to appreciate the important task she will perform tonight.

This year, because the gathering has grown so large, the service has been moved from the cozy chapel to the spacious atrium with soaring ceilings. The room is full of familiar faces: people I met during the first year of grieving are here with their new babies; several, like me, are finally expecting again. It's Dr. Ross's call night, and I wonder if he's stopped by like he did for the fall memorial last year. I scan the room and spot him standing against the wall dressed in scrubs.

Heidi and Beth, who are helping Pat with the service, are waiting to greet me when I walk towards the welcome table.

For Heidi, the first of us to get pregnant again, the past twelve months had been an emotional battle. Her new pregnancy mirrored Brittany's pregnancy on the calendar: both babies were conceived in the month of November, and both were due in the month of August. She was torn between her joy for the new baby and the sorrow of losing

Brittany and continued going to support group meetings throughout her pregnancy, which made her feel guilty, but everyone in group told her it was okay, she was one of them.

After the school year ended in June, she quit her kindergarten teaching job. Now she had more time to take care of herself and more time to worry. At thirty weeks, Heidi panicked because she suddenly couldn't feel the baby move. The nurses quickly found the heartbeat, but Heidi was so shaken that the young doctor on call from her group brought in the ultrasound machine. The baby kicked on screen, but when Heidi insisted she couldn't feel the kicks, he told her maybe she should go see a psychiatrist.

At thirty-two weeks, the point at which Brittany had died, the results of a stress test landed her in the hospital for five days with talk of taking the baby early.

Heidi's anxiety mounted with each passing day. For no clear reason, as she was driving to Beth's one day, she took a different route, one she had never taken before, passing by a stork sign in someone's yard for a baby girl named Kaitlyn Rose. Suddenly her heart swelled. Heidi knew her baby was a girl and had already chosen the name Kaitlyn. Brittany's middle name was Rose. She felt it was a sign from Brittany that everything was going to be okay, that she was watching over her little baby sister from above.

In late July, Heidi—almost to thirty-seven weeks—went into labor. "I'm not staying," Heidi said to the nurse at the hospital when they took her into a delivery room. "You're going to hydrate me and then I'm going home." After waiting so long for this baby, Heidi was in denial that the time had indeed come.

The nurse smiled and when the doctor checked her he said, "Yep, baby day."

Kaitlyn, who was breach, was delivered via c-section while Heidi's mom stood out in the hall with her ear pressed to the operating room door waiting to hear the first cries of her new grandchild.

"Okay, the butt is out," said the doctor.

"I don't hear her crying yet!" panicked Heidi, whose life seemed to be hinging on that first cry.

"It's only her butt!" the doctor said, laughing. He pulled her out, she wailed, Heidi and Greg cried, and it was good.

The next morning while the nurse bathed her, Kaitlyn stopped breathing and turned blue. Being told Kaitlyn had breathing problems triggered the same emotions Heidi had felt more than a year ago when she was told Brittany had died.

After a week in the Neonatal Intensive Care Unit (NICU), and after Heidi and Greg were shown how to do infant CPR, Kaitlyn went home on an apnea monitor which would alert them if she stopped breathing. The alarm went off daily and nightly, sending Heidi into a panic each time she ran into her baby's room. Kaitlyn was also on medicine that made her jittery and cranky. It would be fourteen months before they would be able to take her off the monitor, at which time Heidi promptly threw it out the window.

Beth's pregnancy was not without drama either, beginning with the early onset of uterine contractions. At four months, on her way home from the doctor's office, in the rain, a young driver pulled out in front of her without warning and she smashed into his car. It sent her back to the doctor, but the baby was fine.

Beth immediately put herself on modified bed rest. Up one hour, down two hours. Her doctor managed her symptoms as they arose. Even though she was spotting and contracting just as she had with Josh's pregnancy, she hadn't been diagnosed as having an incompetent cervix because there were no changes in her cervix.

Until she got to twenty weeks.

The doctor was hesitant, but put in a cerclage, a procedure in which a woman's cervix—the opening to the uterus—is stitched shut. But it was done later in the pregnancy than what was usual, and with her cervix already changing and the increased weight of the baby pressing down, the procedure was more difficult. She went home and was put on full bed rest.

Beth and Jeff were broke, and there was no family around to help with two-and-a-half-year-old Madeline. Beth couldn't care for her daughter, but losing another baby was not a price she was willing to pay, even if it meant living on food stamps and credit cards. They found a Montessori school and Jeff took her there every morning and brought her home every evening.

Shortly after, a check arrived in the mail from the insurance company to cover any possible problems Beth might have as a result of the car accident. The $1500 covered the cost of Madeline's Montessori school almost to the penny.

The twenty-four-week mark was a stressful time in the pregnancy; she was nearing the time when she had lost Josh. Still on antidepressants—considered safe at that time, and the OB believing it would be better to continue the medication and avoid another bout with depression—she was calmer than she probably would have been otherwise.

As she approached her due date, they took the cerclage out. The contractions slowly grew steady, she was too excited to sleep, and stayed up all night. In the morning, she went for a walk, and then called the doctor who told her to come in.

When the doctor walked in, she told him her contractions were fifteen minutes apart. "Well fifteen minutes apart isn't going to deliver a baby." Beth broke down crying. "Alright, let me check you." Beth laid back on the examining table. "Oh. You're dilated to five and fully effaced. Okay, I'll send you over to Labor and Delivery."

Jeff's eye widened. "Well, today's really not a good day for me."

Beth almost jumped off the table and choked him. "What do you mean, it's not a good day for you!"

Now in Labor and Delivery, Jeff stood outside in the hall on the phone, trying to change his meetings, and then came into the room and sat down to read the Wall Street Journal. In Jeff's defense, Beth didn't really need his involvement yet; she already had two labor coaches attending to her: Heidi and a friend named Stephanie.

Hours went by. Beth struggled until the epidural took away her pain, and shortly after, she delivered a beautiful, healthy baby girl, Abigail. The room was filled with joy. Beth didn't hope for or expect a boy; she already knew she was having a girl and knowing this gave the baby an identity long before she was born. Beth had her tubes tied afterwards. She couldn't go through another pregnancy again.

Through the delivery and recovery, her focus was on Abigail, but when she left the hospital, it hit her that she had left Josh there more than a year earlier.

I hug Beth and Heidi and ask where the babies are. Both give the same answer: not wanting to cause undue pain to newly bereaved parents, Heidi has left four-month-old Kaitlyn at home with Greg, and Beth has left one-month-old Abigail at home with Jeff.

I pick up a program and scan the rows of seats for two empty chairs, waving to Darlene, Dawn, Wendy, and Tracy who are scattered about. As Alex and I sit down, I glance over at Tracy, trying to gauge her emotional state. Two days after Heidi delivered Kaitlyn, Tracy and Jim were getting ready to leave for their summer vacation in Canada. The doctor's office suggested she come in so they could check on the baby before her trip. Tracy watched for the familiar peanut-shaped form of her developing baby. There on the screen was the baby, but the heartbeat, once beating, was now still. The baby was dead.

Unlike Paul's pregnancy, which had gone to term, this pregnancy had lasted only nine-and-a-half weeks. They hadn't had time to bond with this baby, and Jim's focus had been on the high school baseball team he coached that had just gone to state finals. But Tracy was devastated.

She wasn't yet having any symptoms of miscarriage and they didn't want her to miscarry in Canada. "It could be two months. It could be tomorrow," the doctor told her. Tracy agreed to have a D & C and just like that it was over. They didn't know the sex of the baby, but in her mind it was a girl and they named it Baby Faith. She called her family to tell them she had been pregnant, but now the baby was gone.

They left for Canada, meeting some family there. Tracy was emotionally a wreck and by the time they got home from their road trip, she had a huge blow-out with her sister-in-law that started with a dispute over sandwiches.

When she returned back to work, everyone wanted to know how her vacation was. Nobody knew she had been pregnant until she confided in one friend. Her friend wrote her a letter saying, "You really should tell people because they will support you." She thought about it and decided her friend was right. She couldn't come to work every day pretending her life was fine when inside she felt like she was falling apart all over again.

Last month, on Paul's birthday, Tracy took the day off work, went to church where a mass was being said in Paul's name, ate breakfast at the Omega, and finished with balloons at the cemetery.

She took cupcakes to the support group meeting to celebrate, which must have seemed strange to new attendees, but the veteran group members were all smiling and nodding, knowing full well the importance of celebrating a child's short life.

Wendy is sitting quietly in front of me, alone, letting herself feel the emotions that have been haunting her for so long. Last February, after losing David at sixteen weeks, Wendy made herself wait six long months before trying to conceive. Her doctor did genetic studies on baby David, Mark, and Wendy, and although the studies ruled out many possibilities, they were inconclusive as to why she was having trouble.

She was thirty-five, Michael was three, and the closeness of her baby's ages was important to her. "Do we have to do this? Can't we just let it happen?" Mark asked.

"No, I have a window. I need another baby. Time is wasting," Wendy pleaded. She found herself pregnant immediately.

Last month, almost ten weeks into her pregnancy, Wendy prepared to have a cerclage put in, hoping to keep the cervix closed and prevent the circumstances that forced David into the world too early. But first the doctor sent Wendy for an ultrasound to date the baby according to size. She went alone after work. *This is going to turn out alright. This needs to be okay,* she told herself. Sitting outside the ultrasound room waiting, she broke into a nervous sweat. *This doesn't have to turn out. This might not turn out.*

Once inside, she waited expectantly for the results. "The sac is empty. It's a blighted ovum," said the ultrasound tech.

"There was a baby there. I saw it!" Wendy insisted, remembering the earlier ultrasounds she had done while on nursing duty. She was overcome with grief, too numb to even cry. It felt as if someone had kicked her in the chest. As she processed the reality of yet another loss, the anger washed over her. She honestly believed all she needed to do was ask and it would be given to her. *The Lord takes care of us.* If she prayed hard enough, if she wanted it bad enough, it had to turn out. She couldn't understand why this kept happening to her, to her babies.

This time she had to call her friend Marianne in the nursery to come down and be with her. As Marianne drove Wendy home, Wendy called her mom from the car. Wendy's mom answered the phone amidst a party for Wendy's sister-in-law. "Mom, I lost another baby."

"Not another one!" Her mom was always there physically, but when it came to emotional support, Wendy still felt a void in her relationship with her mom, whose reaction to Wendy's third loss seemed callous, and harsh. Wendy felt guilty, as if her mother was annoyed that Wendy's news was putting a damper on the party. Again, Wendy felt alone. So alone. Why wasn't somebody there enfolding her in their arms and saying this is the worst thing that could ever happen? she wondered. As she traveled down the Dan Ryan expressway out of Chicago with another dead baby in her womb, she felt as if she were living out a never-ending bad dream.

She waited for days for her body to miscarry her baby; she couldn't yet grieve because there was no closure. Finally, unable to bear the waiting, she took matters into her own hands, scheduling a D & C with her doctor who had delivered Michael and performed the first

D & C with Kelly. Mark went with her. The residents did their job as
if it were just another procedure, *easy come, easy go.* Wendy felt as
though she weren't even there. She named this baby Hope. Her journal entry was as brief as the baby's life.

> *November 23, 1996*
>   *Trick. Lost a third baby. Nine, almost ten weeks.*
> *They called you a "blighted ovum." I saw you at seven weeks.*
> *You were there.*

Why can't I just be satisfied with my one child? Wendy tortured
herself. Feelings of guilt plagued her, but Wendy knew the closeness of
a sibling and wanted desperately for Michael to know that, too.

    She was still hopeful about a baby and wouldn't give up.
Nobody told her she couldn't have a baby. They just didn't know why
she kept losing them. The doctors didn't know what to do for her. It
was like someone telling you your child is sick, but they don't know
why and don't know what to do. These were her children; she had to
fix what was broken.

    After losing Hope, she couldn't bear to go back to work in the
hospital's infant nursery and was assigned to the cardiac rehab floor.
She also left behind her work on a committee to improve the
procedures for dealing with premature deliveries.

    Tonight, as families take turns putting ornaments on the
Christmas tree in the front of the room, one for each of their lost
babies, Wendy is mortified that she holds three angel ornaments in her
hand. Someone has brought a baby, and the baby is crying, which
makes her pain that much sharper.

    I whisper in Alex's ear that it's time, and she takes my hand and
pulls me up to the tree, proudly hanging her baby sister's angel among
the others.

    After Beth and Heidi hand out their handmade angel keep-
sakes and the last song trails off, the seven of us congregate in the back

of the room. Dr. Ross is nowhere in sight, and I assume he's been called back to the Birth Center to deliver a baby.

Beth invites us all to her house for a visit. Looking at Alex who's as tired as I am, I reluctantly decline. But not before Darlene has a chance to tell everyone she's seven weeks pregnant. I've been wondering all these months. She told us last year that although she wasn't emotionally ready for a new pregnancy, she wasn't preventing it. Everyone surrounds Darlene for a big group hug.

"So, I hope you get a good employee discount at the Baby Superstore," I tell Darlene.

"Actually," she says, "I don't work there anymore. I just got a new job at The Baby's Room."

"Another baby store?" Heidi asks, laughing.

"Yeah, I guess you were overdue for a new job," says Beth.

This is Darlene's second baby store gig in eight months, her fourth baby-related job since losing the twins.

"I already know what I want," says Darlene. "When I showed Larry the expensive crib and angel bedding I want to buy for the new baby with my employee discount, Larry shook his head. He's afraid the solid oak crib that converts to a toddler bed is so heavy it might fall through the floor of our apartment."

This makes us all laugh. Even Dawn, who's had a long, unfruitful year, can't help but laugh over Larry's crib veto.

After Dawn's miscarriage last December, she began to believe she and Andy would never have children of their own. With no job and no baby, she was completely lost. "I don't know what to do anymore," she told Andy. Insurance didn't cover in-vitro fertilization (IVF), which cost up to $10,000 each time. They began questioning everything. Do we find another doctor? Do we give up on this and try to adopt? She knew she was capable of becoming pregnant and didn't want to give up hope.

They found a new infertility doctor, one with a different attitude. "You're not going to be a success until you have a baby in your arms," he told them.

After failed insemination attempts, the doctor did his best to surgically remove the large clump of adhesions that were discovered on Dawn's uterus, ovaries, and Fallopian tubes. He told her IVF was her only hope for pregnancy, and they've scheduled the procedure for January, giving Dawn time to get through the holidays and have her annual checkup with her OB.

~ ~ ~

As I drive home, I slide my hand over my growing belly and glance in the rearview mirror at Alex. Tonight, I feel blessed as I bask in the goodness and abundance of life. Tonight, my hope in the future outweighs the uncertainty and fear I've felt for so long, and as a soft snow begins to fall, I wonder how long it will be before Dawn, Tracy, and Wendy share in the joy Heidi, Beth, Darlene, and I feel.

26

As 1996 comes to a close, my Christmas holiday is not only survived, but filled once again with hope. Although my focus is on Alex and the new life growing inside, Miranda is never far from my thoughts. While Alex and Al help me unpack Christmas ornaments to decorate the freshly cut pine tree standing naked in the family room, Alex pulls out a white box with candy cane swirls that holds the few ornaments I have for Miranda: an odd assortment of angels and teddy bears that were given as gifts last year, some for Miranda and some Miranda has inherited from me. For the few minutes Alex and I hang them on the tree, I am misty-eyed and missing my child who would be eighteen months old now—just big enough to make a mess of everything and pull the ornaments off the tree quicker than we can get them up. The feeling quickly passes as Alex squeals at the sight of the electric train Daddy has just pulled out.

Determined to do something meaningful regarding Miranda this year, I filled her stocking with gifts we could then donate to a child in need. My plan backfires when Alex asks why Santa doesn't know Miranda is in heaven, and since her sister isn't here to play with the toys, can she keep them?

Drifting into January and a new year—1997—I come home from the book store with an Anne Geddes baby photo calendar and coffee table book. By surrounding myself with happy images of babies,

I'm hoping to remember that pregnancy and childbirth don't always end in heartbreak.

I'm not the only one who will need the same reassurance. In December, just after the memorial service, Dawn was at her OB's office for a check-up and mentioned her period was one week late. Although this was not unusual, she wondered if she possibly could be pregnant, even though her new infertility specialist told her it wouldn't happen on its own.

"You're pregnant!" said the nurse a few minutes after giving Dawn a pregnancy test. Dawn looked at her with disbelief. This wasn't something to joke about with a woman who had lost triplets.

"I'm telling you, you're pregnant. It's faint, but you're pregnant."

Dawn was still glaring at the nurse when the doctor walked in. "Let's send you home with another test to do in one week." That week seemed like forever to Dawn. She waited until late one night so she could leave it for Andy to find early the next morning, but he was awake and knew full well what Dawn was doing in the bathroom. "Well, what is it?" he yelled to her from the bedroom. She walked out of the bathroom and looked at him.

"It's positive," she said, still in disbelief. But there it was, a big red plus sign, as plain as could be. "I don't know how this happened," she said. "I mean, I know how it happened, but it just can't be. They said it doesn't happen. It just couldn't have happened. I guess all I needed was a little Roto-Rooter on the inside, and now I'm as good as new. Suddenly the plumbing works."

The next day, a blood test confirmed Dawn was indeed pregnant. She called her infertility office. "I don't think I'll be coming in to do that IVF cycle in January."

"Well, is there a problem?"

"I'm pregnant!" she blurted out, no longer able to contain her excitement.

"We need to see you right away to do some blood work," they told her.

It was Christmas Eve. Dawn had been stuck with a needle seven times in two days to confirm she was pregnant. "Let's not get excited about this," the infertility doctor told her, "because I'm afraid this might be a tubal pregnancy." *Well, thank you for raining on my parade right now,* Dawn thought to herself, *while I'm sitting here calling you a miracle worker.*

"I normally don't like to do this during the holidays, but let's find out right now," he said. He performed an ultrasound to determine the location of the implanted egg. "It's in the uterus. It's right where it should be!" he said pointing to a spot on the screen that appeared to blink on and off. It was the beating of a tiny heart. They still couldn't believe what their eyes saw. "Let's be very cautious," he warned them, putting her on hormone supplements and giving her a list of restrictions. Unlike her former infertility doctor who waved goodbye at the first sign of conception, this doctor would follow her through the first thirteen weeks of pregnancy.

For Christmas they gave cards to their family members with an ultrasound picture of the growing baby and a handwritten message saying, "Didn't know what to get you for Christmas…it's due to be here in August." Andy's mom opened up the picture before reading the card and stared down at it with a strange look on her face. "You know what that is, don't you?" Dawn asked.

"It's a picture of the triplets?" Andy's mom answered in disbelief.

"No," Dawn said.

"Oh my God!" shouted everyone when they realized what they were looking at. "And it happened without any intervention," Dawn added.

"So this is the real thing," someone commented, implying the triplets weren't real because medical technology had helped bring them into the world. Dawn was too overwhelmed with joy to be annoyed.

~ ~ ~

A few weeks later, I receive a call from Heidi with news about Tracy. When Tracy miscarried Faith last July, she was thirty-eight years old and desperate to be a mother. She and Jim had recently moved into a larger house with plenty of rooms for children, a big backyard to play in, and the elementary school across the street. By September, they began trying to conceive. She knew the right days, and every time her period came she was more devastated. She was having sinus problems and seemed to be at the doctor's office every month, answering "no" every time they asked her if she was pregnant before giving her a new medication.

After the Christmas memorial service, they left for a vacation in Montana. Her period was late, and she and Jim drove all over the middle of nowhere until they found a pharmacy and bought a pregnancy test. "You know," Jim said, "why don't you wait until we get home to take the test because you'll just be disappointed." She agreed and packed it away in her suitcase.

When they returned from their trip, Tracy went straight to the doctor for her sinus problem. "When was your last period?" the doctor asked.

"Actually, I'm late," Tracy answered.

"It could be because of your sinus infection."

"Well, we are trying to get pregnant."

"I want to give you a new antibiotic, but let's just do a pregnancy test first." Tracy waited, knowing the woman was wasting her time. She came out with a beaming smile. "Tracy, you're pregnant!" Tracy sat in a moment of disbelief. She couldn't contain her excitement and called Jim from work.

"You will not believe it! We're pregnant! You should have let me take the test in Montana!" But now she worried the medications she was taking could have harmed the developing baby.

Tracy was due in August, one week after Dawn. And like Dawn, Tracy's pregnancy brought a mix of emotions. She counted the days leading up to nine weeks, the point at which she had suffered the miscarriage. Getting past that day was good. But she had lost Paul at the end with no warning and no reason, and it was difficult to ignore the very real possibility that she could carry this baby to term and lose it the same way. She forced the thoughts out of her head, refusing to dwell on something she had no control over.

~ ~ ~

A few days later, I get another phone call, this time from Beth. It's about Darlene. At eleven weeks, Darlene's cervix began to shorten. The doctor put in a cerclage, and two days later she was in bed with a fever and cold sweats. She thought she had the flu; the doctor feared infection. By the third day, she had a pink-tinged discharge and pain every seven minutes so strong she was pounding her fist on the side of the car as Larry drove her to the doctor's office.

An ultrasound confirmed the baby still had a heartbeat and everything looked fine, so the doctor on call sent her home with antibiotics and told her to rest. The pain worsened on the drive home, and as Larry parked the car, Darlene felt a warm gush between her legs. She rushed into the bathroom and onto the toilet, blood and amniotic fluid everywhere. Just a few days ago, the doctor had told her the cerclage would keep the baby inside, dead or alive.

When she looked down, she saw her baby floating in the toilet.

Her legs went limp, and as she slumped towards the floor sobbing, Larry grabbed her and set her down gently. "My baby's dead, another baby is dead," she cried. Larry turned around and punched a hole through the wall.

She got on the phone with the doctor's office. "You just told me everything is fine. I want to know, if everything is fine, then why is my baby dead in the toilet?" she cried. They told her to come back to the office. "I'm not coming in. I'm not coming to your office!" They told her they needed to check her and possibly do a D & C. "You don't understand, my husband punched a hole in the wall. He probably needs to go to the hospital now too, and if he sees the doctor he'll probably punch the doctor." They told her to come anyway. "I'm not coming in until my regular doctor is in the office." They told her he was interviewing residents and wouldn't be in until tomorrow. "Then I'll wait until tomorrow." They told her she needed to collect the baby out of the toilet and put it in a bowl.

"Larry you have to do this. I can't do it," Darlene told him.

Larry was crying. "I can't believe I have to do this." He reached down with a bowl and scooped out the three-inch form. She couldn't tell if the baby was a boy or a girl, but it had fingers and toes, a nose, mouth, and ears, and a tiny cord still attached to a piece of placenta.

She got back on the phone. "It's all in one piece and in a bowl of water right now, what do I do?"

"Just leave it how it is, try to find a lid and bring it in with you."

"Do I bring it in like this? Or do I bring it in a lunch bag? How do I conceal it so no one knows I'm walking around with a dead baby?"

"Put it in a bag."

She laid down to rest, and it wasn't long before Larry convinced her to make the forty-minute trip back to the office. She sat in the waiting room for thirty minutes with the bag on her lap, watching pregnant teenagers walk in and out. Darlene asked if there was another room she could wait in where there weren't pregnant people, but they told her, "Sorry, no."

Finally in an exam room, she was surprised and relieved when her doctor walked in. "They told me you weren't here," she said.

"Yeah, they told me what was going on and I wanted to be here. How are you?" he asked.

"I'm fine," she answered.

"No, you're not, you just lost your baby."

The painful exam confirmed that her body hadn't expelled all of the tissue, and she was taken up to the hospital Labor and Delivery floor for a D & C. As she was wheeled into an operating room, she listened to the cries of a newborn baby who had just been delivered across the hall. "I'm sorry, Darlene," her doctor told her. Later, Larry saw the doctor sitting at the desk with his head down, face in his hands, another doctor consoling him.

A few days later, after an autopsy, the doctor's office called to say they had Darlene's baby. This time she knew what to do and told them she wanted to see and baptize her baby. Beth and Heidi met them at the hospital. The chaplain pointed out the baby looked like a boy, so they named him Andrew, dipped their fingers into a seashell filled with holy water, and baptized him one drop at a time. After emptying the water, they placed Andrew in the seashell, taking pictures as they passed him around to each other.

The chaplain took Andrew to a funeral home for cremation, and his remains were put in a wooden urn with a carving of an angel holding a baby. Darlene moved the remains of Nathan and Nicholas, each kept in separate bags, from their plain box to the new urn with their younger brother.

As the weeks went by, Darlene felt twitches in her stomach, like a kicking baby, and started to believe that maybe she had been carrying twins again and one was still alive. But the ultrasound would have shown another baby and the D & C scraped the inside of her uterus clean. Still, she couldn't shake the feeling.

Shortly after, an unexpected package arrived in the mail. Larry's aunt had sent a care package: gift certificates for a massage and manicure, bath salts, a healing book, cookies, and tea. The surprise wasn't so much the package as who it had come from; the woman was known as an all-about-me person.

Emotionally a mess, Darlene started taking birth control pills. But every pill she took was crushing because she was forcing herself not to have a family when it was all she could think about, and a month later she threw out the pills. "If it happens, it happens," she told Larry.

27

At twenty weeks, I begin to feel my baby's subtle kicks and rolls: a blessing when the baby is active, a curse when the baby is still.

At work and on the street, I field questions daily: do I know if I'm having a boy or a girl, and do I have a name picked out? I tell people I'm fairly sure the baby is a girl, and no, we haven't chosen a name yet. Most are disappointed when I deny them the chance to critique my name choices. What I don't tell them is that I often catch myself calling this baby Miranda.

In my mind, it's much too early to think about baby names. We still have so far to go yet, and anything could go wrong. While talking to some friends at church about stillbirth, they each tell me about recent full-term cord accidents they know about. I put on a brave face while my heart sinks. I know what the statistics are. The chances are slim, but I could experience another cord accident. I force it out of my mind. There's nothing I can do.

Dr. Ross follows through on his earlier promise to send me for a level II ultrasound, "just to make sure." There's no medical indication anything is wrong with this pregnancy, but given my history, nobody is going to question my motives. I'm hesitant to tell the radiologist why I'm really here. I want to know if an ultrasound could have saved Miranda, and will we be able to detect an umbilical cord problem with this baby? When I finally tell him my history, I expect to be treated like just another over-anxious expectant mother. But he seems to understand my anxiety and answers my questions with honesty and respect. He tells us that even had we performed an ultrasound during Miranda's pregnancy, we might not have detected a problem. The limitations of this technology make it impossible to see every section of the cord. Having always wondered *What if?* his answer helps put my mind at ease once and for all. Everything looks perfect with this baby and the cord, as accurately as he can tell.

He asks if I want to know the sex, and although I'm sure I already know the answer, I nod my head. With about ninety-five percent sureness, he tells us we're going to have a girl. I smile up at Al who squeezes my hand. "But if it turns out to be a boy, don't send me the bill from Talbot's for little pink outfits," he adds.

~ ~ ~

On February 18th, I look at my calendar and a little voice reminds me today is the anniversary of David's death. When I call Wendy to see how she's doing, I can tell by the tone in her voice the answer is not good. "I'm off today, why don't I come down with Alex for a visit?" I ask her.

"Really?" she says. "That would be great. Michael will love having someone to play with, too."

Over salad and sandwiches, Wendy tells me she's thinking about joining a prayer group at church. She was still going to the support group, but her attendance had started to become sporadic. There was only so much she could talk about, and after a while she had said it all. She found it increasingly difficult to make the forty-five-minute drive to the hospital and come home late, emotionally drained, and several of us had already stopped going to meetings.

When I finally pull Alex away from playing with her new friend and get her to the door, I hug Wendy tight. "Thanks for lunch. It was great."

"Oh, stop it. It was nothing. I'm glad you came down."

"I'm glad too," I smile. "Maybe we can meet at a park when it warms up."

"Yeah."

"Hang in there, okay?"

"Oh, I will," she answers.

As I pull away, I wave, wishing I didn't have to leave Wendy alone, and wishing I didn't live forty-five minutes away.

~ ~ ~

That night, Wendy turned once again to her journal.

February 18, 1997
Dear David,

I went to the flower shop this afternoon hoping to find something to put on your grave. Only, nothing seems appropriate because I feel as though I shouldn't be visiting your grave. I should be holding you. You would be about six months old—a wonderful age—full of smiles and baby babble. I imagine you to be like Michael, maybe curly blond hair and perhaps a bit more energetic. Your big brother was such a "calm" baby, easy to fall into a schedule, adaptable. People warned me that my next child was going to give me a go. I was kind of frightened of that because I'm impatient. Maybe I wouldn't have treated you the best. I feel like God knows that about me and called you back to Him.

It hurts so much to never have had you. I cling to "things" that I have assigned to you, hoping never to forget you: like yellow. It speaks to me of sun, wild flowers, warmth and happiness. Another color that is yours is purple—deep, unforgiven, unrelenting, passionate, heart beating. And dear little one, the teddy bear I've named Davee—soft, mine, has in my heart become my pseudo baby. Surprisingly, I admitted that a couple of nights ago to the support group. It was memory night. I look for teddy bear cards for your scrapbook. I listen for songs I yearn to sing to you. The lullabies I sang for Michael are bittersweet. Beautiful memories of Michael. Empty air for you. Should I sing them for you? I get stuck in the pain.

Six months old. I remember I needed to change the infant car seat to the bigger one for Michael when he was this age. Would you have been as big? Where are you now? Will you bring me back to Him? Is this pity/grief useless? I wish I had a song in my head for you. What comes to mind is

"Baby mine, close your eyes
Rest your head close to my heart
Never to part
Baby of mine"
How about this one
"Sunshine on the water makes me happy
Sunshine in my eyes can make me smile"
Did He know you were my sunshine?

I dread the night, especially tonight. A year ago tomorrow you left me. David, if I could only find peace with not understanding why, then I would give up this self-torture.
"Give it to the Lord."
"Lord you know my heart and its ways, you who formed me before I was born.
In the secret of darkness before I saw the sun
In my mother's womb."

~ ~ ~

Dr. Ross assumes I will want another c-section. I'm hoping to avoid surgery and with it, a long, difficult recovery. But there are risks with a vaginal birth after c-section (VBAC) and I'm not willing to take any risks with this baby. After lengthy discussion, we agree: A c-section birth will be the quickest, safest way to deliver my long-awaited baby.

He pulls out a calendar. "I want you to get to at least thirty-eight weeks. Pick any Monday, May 12th or after."

"Isn't Monday your day off?" I ask.

"Yes."

"Don't you want to schedule it for a Thursday when you're on call?"

"No, I want to be able to give you my full attention. I don't want to be delivering any other babies."

I smile and tell him May 12th will be perfect.

Besides the obvious fact that I can't wait to hold my new baby, I look forward to leaving my job and, once again, have been counting down: eight weeks of work, ten until my delivery. My department's upcoming reorganization is leaving me without a position, and instead of putting in for a transfer, I've decided to say goodbye. I've grown tired of juggling the demands of home and work, children and bosses. It had never been a fulfilling career for me, but merely a job to pay some bills and provide insurance. I've learned that life is too short, too unpredictable, and I have to make choices, do the things that make me happy, spend time with the people I love the most. Alex is growing up so fast, and I don't know how much time I'll be given to be her mother; I don't want to miss a moment.

~ ~ ~

The closer I get to my due date, the less the baby moves. Each night I lie in bed waiting for some sign of life, praying for just one little kick. As each minute ticks by, the worry builds that something has happened to my baby, that she's gone. It happened so easily with Miranda. Each time I'm ready to pick up the phone and tell Dr. Ross I'm coming in, the baby moves. I anxiously count the days until my next appointment and pray to God to keep this baby safe until May 12th.

Now that I'm going in for weekly visits, the Gestapo office manager sternly asks if I've seen the other doctors yet, and I dodge the question. I don't see the point in wasting my time with the other doctors. They don't know me or my history. I'm at a critical time now and need extra TLC, and unless something unexpected happens, Dr. Ross is going to deliver my baby.

Near my last day of work, my coworkers have a going away party for me. I won't miss my job, but I will miss my dear friends, especially Lynne.

~ ~ ~

With my first two pregnancies, the excitement and anticipation had gotten the best of me: I stocked up on diapers and baby bath, and washed and folded baby clothes months before my due date. But now, well, I know the pain of having to put away those things no longer needed for a baby who will never come home. I can't bear to do it again should something go wrong and have decided to wait until the last possible moment.

During the past few days, I've washed only things I'll need assuming I bring the baby home with me this time, keeping it to a bare minimum: some one-piece underwear, a few lightweight sleepers, several receiving blankets, burp cloths, and one crib sheet. I've bought one package of diapers and one package of wipes.

I'm fooling myself by thinking I can shut off the emotions of hope and excitement for this baby. I tell myself that if I don't prepare and don't get attached, I'll be spared the devastation. The reality is if this baby dies too, I'll be just as devastated anyway. I'm already attached.

~ ~ ~

The night before my delivery, I retreat into the bathroom, light several candles and slide into the bathtub. Excited and scared, I know I won't be able to truly relax until my baby is in my arms, alive and well. *This is it,* I think as I take a deep breath. *Please God, I pray, please let everything go well tomorrow. Please let my baby be okay.* I know prayer didn't save all of my friends' babies, but it's all I have.

28

I get no sleep. Back pain and anxiety about the surgery keep me awake most of the night. Al's parents come early in the morning to take care of Alex, and we arrive at the hospital by 6:30 a.m. I catch a glimpse of Dr. Ross down the hall. He looks tired. One of the nurses whispers to me he's been here all weekend. My heart sinks. I imagined him arriving early, fresh from a restful weekend. She hands a pair of scrubs to Al, tells him he can change down the hall, and takes me into a room to prep me for surgery by shaving my belly, inserting a catheter, and beginning an IV. Dr. Ross walks in, shakes hands with Al, and comes over and puts his hand on my shoulder, smiling down at me.

"You're not too tired for this, are you?" I ask, trying to hide my anxiety while visions of him falling asleep and dropping the scalpel into my uterus race through my mind.

"No, I'm fine. How are you?" he asks.

"A little nervous," I answer with a forced smile.

"I know. I'm going to do everything in my power to get the baby out safe and sound and into your arms as quickly as possible."

He asks the nurse if Dr. Jones is here. "Not yet," she answers.

"We'll be ready to go as soon as the anesthesiologist gets here," he tells me.

"I thought Dr. Berg was scheduled to do my epidural," I remind him. Wanting to surround me with people who would understand my loss and be more sensitive to my needs, Dr. Ross had requested Dr. Berg because he and his wife had also lost their baby girl shortly after us two years ago.

"Dr. Berg's wife just had a baby. He's up on the maternity floor with her right now."

"Oh," I answer, disappointed Dr. Berg is unavailable. Then the news sinks in, and I smile. "Okay, I guess he deserves the day off."

I'm wheeled into the cold, bright operating room, and Dr. Ross and his nurses lift me onto the narrow operating table. I feel as if I might roll right off, and I begin to shiver uncontrollably, perhaps more from nerves than from the chilly air. They see me shaking and cover me with warm blankets. "Are you ready?" asks Dr. Jones.

"Yes." I roll onto my side and ask the nurse to hold my hand while the epidural needle goes in. Then I'm rolled onto my back, legs strapped down, and ask for oxygen before the room starts to spin. The operating room is beginning to hustle and bustle, with masked faces coming in and out, moving about getting instruments ready. Al sits by my side holding my hand. My other arm is outstretched on a board with a pulse monitor taped to my finger. A tall man wearing a mask comes over and introduces himself. "Hi Mr. and Mrs. Novak, I'm Dr. Fitzgerald, the neonatologist." Worried thoughts fill my head. Why is he here? I don't remember a neonatologist being at Alex's delivery. Is something wrong that they aren't telling me about? As if reading my mind, he explains that a neonatologist is now present at all c-section births as a precaution.

"Monica, let me know if you feel anything," says Dr. Ross as he begins poking my belly in different places. I feel nothing. "Okay, I'm going to start the incision now. You shouldn't feel any pain, but if you do let me know right away." I remain calm, staring up at the ceiling and focusing on my breathing. The incision takes only minutes. Then the familiar tugging begins. It doesn't hurt, but I feel a crushing weight in my chest and, gasping for breath, I start to panic.

"I can't breathe!"

"Try to relax," says Dr. Ross, "the baby is pushing on your lungs. We'll have her out in a minute."

Why is this taking so long? Doesn't she want to come out? Suddenly, the pressure inside me is gone and I suck in a deep breath. "Here she is!" the nurse announces. "She's beautiful, look at those eyelashes!" The emotions that have been deep inside me for so long come pouring out, and I begin crying hysterically. I smile over at Al as he touches my cheek and squeezes my hand. I get a glimpse of my baby as they carry her over to a warming table, and Al gets up to follow her.

I realize she isn't crying. *Oh my God, something's wrong. She's supposed to be crying.* Still flat on the table while Dr. Ross stitches my incision, I struggle to look over my shoulder at her, but my eyes are still filled with tears. "Why isn't she crying?" I yell in a panic.

"Mrs. Novak, your baby is alright," answers Dr. Fitzgerald. "The reason you don't hear her crying is because she has some fluid in her lungs and we're suctioning it out. It happens in about 50% of all c-section births."

Al comes back over and sits by my side. "Is she okay?" I ask him. "She's fine. She's beautiful."

"Seven pounds, eight ounces," a nurse calls out.

"When can I hold her?" I ask.

"We're going to have to take her up to the Neonatal Intensive Care Unit to give her some oxygen. You can come see her as soon as you feel able," says Dr. Fitzgerald, and they wheel her away.

In recovery, I sit half propped, nervously popping ice chips in my mouth. I haven't eaten since last night and my stomach is protesting. I know the routine: ice chips for twenty-four hours, then clear liquids until I pass gas. "I can't believe this is happening," I complain to Al. "I've waited so long for this, and now I can't even hold her."

"I know," he sympathizes. Three recoveries, all bad. The first time, something had gone wrong with my epidural pump, and I had been in too much pain to hold Alex, reluctantly sending her to the nursery. The second time, I held my dead baby. This time was supposed to be perfect. As my baby lies under an oxygen hood on the third floor, it's less than perfect. But she's alive and otherwise healthy, and I'm grateful for that.

As soon as I get settled into my room on the third floor, I ask to go see the baby. Al pushes my wheelchair down the hall and up to the door of the NICU. I ring the doorbell and wait for a nurse to let us in. She instructs us to wash our hands at the sink just inside the door, and we follow her into the large open room. Expecting a dark, quiet atmosphere, I'm surprised by the commotion. The room is brightly lit, busy nurses rushing back and forth checking on beeping monitors that seem to go off every thirty seconds. Almost every bassinet and incubator has an occupant. There must be twelve other babies here. We ask a nurse to show us where the Novak baby is. She takes us around a bank of bassinets to the corner of the room near a window.

Al wheels me close. "She has to stay under the oxygen hood," the nurse explains, "but you can touch her and hold her hands."

"Oh, look at her," I cry. "She looks so helpless." Casey is asleep on her back, wearing only a diaper, the heat lamp above keeping her warm, a clear plastic oxygen hood sitting over her head. Wires attached to her body, four from her chest, one from her left toe, snake around and lead up to the blinking monitors above, and an IV is taped to her right leg. I don't know what any of these things are doing, and for the moment I don't care. I just want to hold my baby. I reach over and wrap my fingers around her tiny hand. She's so beautiful, so perfect. Her head is covered with dark hair, her skin a healthy pink glow. And, yes, she does have those long eyelashes like both her sisters did. I stroke her tiny, soft feet, and as I turn and smile at Al, he snaps a picture of us. Casey's first picture. As I watch my baby sleep peacefully, I suddenly realize how tired I am. She's content and in good hands, so Al takes me back to my room to rest.

My parents arrive and after long hugs, we explain the baby's situation. "What's her name?" my dad asks.

"Oh, it's Casey. Well, Cassandra, but we'll call her Casey." It wasn't until my final trimester that I began to bug Al about baby names. He also had protected himself with a wait-and-see attitude about the baby, but I didn't want to leave this important decision until the last minute and then regret my lack of planning. The name Samantha was also still at the top of our list, and I agonized over it for weeks. While lying in bed one night, I turned to a higher power, asking God to let me know which name I should give to this precious child.

During the next few weeks, I received my answer. I took a phone message for my sister-in-law from a young woman named Casey. The same day, I saw a character on a video named Casey. In the same week, I heard two female radio callers named Casey. The name walked by me on a shopping bag at Alex's preschool. I accidentally came upon Casey, Illinois on an atlas and the next day drove past Casey's Auto Shop. Finally, a woman at the park was calling her dog— Casey. It wasn't a common name, and what at first appeared to be coincidence soon became a message I could no longer deny. We agreed on the name Cassandra; Casey for short.

"Great, now I have two granddaughters with boy's names," my dad teases.

"Well, it's the closest I could get you to a grandson," I shoot back with a grin.

The door opens and a bunch of balloons walk in. Behind the balloons is my dear friend, Lucy, from church. Visiting hours don't start until 2:00 and I haven't called anyone yet, so I'm surprised to see her. "I talked my way in," she laughs and gives me a big hug. "I'm so happy for you." She starts to cry, which makes me start to cry. Lucy didn't know me when Miranda died, but I remember the day I told her the story while we painted the church nursery and shared the joys and sorrows of our lives. "I love you," I tell her, hugging her back. "I love you too. I'm not going to stay. You look tired. But I'll be back."

Al makes several trips back to the nursery with Alex and her grandparents. With nurses and techs in and out of my room, and phone calls from friends and family, I get no rest for the remainder of the day.

Dr. Fitzgerald, "Fitz" as he's known around here, tells us Casey is doing fine, but she needs to stay under the oxygen hood for at least twenty-four hours. She's also being given antibiotics to prevent infection, such as pneumonia. Although her condition is not critical, I feel better knowing she's in good hands. Dr. Fitz is a cutting-edge neonatologist who in 1989 cared for the smallest surviving baby born alive who was later featured in the Guinness Book of World Records.

"When can we hold her?" I ask.

"After we take the oxygen hood off, probably some time tomorrow," he answers. My heart sinks.

Beth and Heidi come in that evening with gifts for Casey and Alex. Several friends from church follow them in, and my large, private room suddenly feels like a party closet. We're breaking maternity floor policy by having so many visitors in my room, but perhaps knowing my history, the nurses let it slide. Pat Vaci comes in and gives us a handful of Polaroids she's taken of Casey, and Al tapes one to the box of "It's a Girl" chocolate cigars. Pat's well known around here for her Polaroids. The hospital gave her an award for compassion after she snapped a Polaroid of a critically ill baby minutes before he was airlifted to another hospital so the baby's parents, who were left behind, would have a photo of him.

~ ~ ~

I sit in my room alone the next morning, missing Casey who seems so far down the hall, and missing Miranda who feels a million miles from earth. I slowly get out of bed, walk over to the small round table across the room and pick up the white leather photo album with flowers etched on the cover.

Miranda's photos, including the Polaroids that took me six months to ask my dad for, and mementos had been sitting in a box hidden in my closet for nearly two years. Just weeks ago, as Casey's delivery date approached, Beth, a former Creative Memories™ consultant, taught a scrapbooking workshop for parents who had lost a baby. I finished the first page at the workshop and was on my way to putting together an entire book.

The week before my delivery, I worked on the scrapbook every day while Alex was at preschool or otherwise occupied. Materials were spread out all over the family room floor while I worked at the kitchen table with my scissors, glue, colored pens, and a tissue box; I cried the entire time. Miranda's short life unfolded before me as the pages were filled with photos, poems, cards, certificates, her hospital bracelet, baptismal gown, and a lock of her hair. Throughout the book, I copied down quotes I had found during my first year of grieving that I turned to whenever I became weighed down by the emptiness and despair—words from other bereaved parents that brought me comfort and gave me hope. Finally, just days before Casey's birth, I added the final piece to Miranda's book, a saying I cut out of a baby memory booklet, *Little Footprints* by Dorothy Ferguson, that Candy had given me two years earlier in the hospital:

As your parents, we will never sign school papers or see your name on pictures that decorate our refrigerator. The special things kept here mark your life and death. Your little footprints have placed a signature on our hearts like no other ever will.

When Alex came home that day, I called her to sit down next to me on the couch, struggling to find the words to begin, unsure of what her reaction would be. We often talked about Miranda, but she was seeing these pictures for the first time. This was the only tangible proof of her baby sister's existence, and not surprisingly, she had many questions, which I answered as simply and honestly as I could. No longer able to hide my tears, I hugged Alex, tried to explain why I was crying and finished off the tissue box.

I settle back into bed and open the cover of Miranda's book.

Miranda Blair Novak
June 20, 1995
Forever in Our Hearts

As I turn the page and look at her photograph, tears stream down my face. Opposite is a picture of me towards the end of her pregnancy, happy and carefree, excited and naïve.

Emotions wash over me and I break down sobbing. I've waited so long to have a baby, almost three years since I got pregnant with Miranda. For the past nine months, when I wasn't envisioning a dead baby, I imagined lounging in my room cuddling and nursing my baby. Now I'm alone and helpless, and all of the memories and sorrow of losing Miranda have come flooding back, details as vivid as if it happened yesterday. I suddenly miss her now more than I have in months, remembering all of the things I missed as her mother: holding, rocking, nursing, singing, looking into her eyes, playing with her fingers.

I call Pat whose office is down the hall. She comes quickly and sits down next to my bed, taking my hand in hers and listening intently as I cry about Casey and Miranda. When I've finally calmed down, Pat asks if she can see the book in my lap. Tears stream down her face as she turns the pages.

Over the years, I've come to learn Pat does much more than facilitate a support group for bereaved parents. When she's not supporting women in high-risk pregnancies and families whose babies are critically ill, or counseling parents through pregnancy and infant loss, or educating staff about the needs of these special people, or snapping Polaroids, she's sitting with mothers who can't make up their minds about whether to be happy about the birth of the new baby or distraught over the death of the previous one.

"This is beautiful."

"It only took me two years to finally do it," I say, trying to laugh.

"That's okay. And it's okay to feel sad right now."

"I miss Casey so much, I haven't even gotten to hold her yet."

"Would you like to go down and see her?" Pat asks. I nod. She holds out her arm for me to grab as I slowly pull myself out of bed, and we make the walk down the long hallway. When we get to Casey's corner of the nursery, Pat pulls up a chair for me. My heart sinks upon seeing the oxygen hood over her head. I had been hoping it would be off by now so that I could hold her. One of the nurses comes over and tells me Casey knocked her oxygen hood onto the floor during the night, quickly earning the nickname "Feisty" from the NICU staff. Pat and I laugh in disbelief. I can't wait to tell Al how strong and spirited our little girl is already.

As I stroke her hand, Dr. Fitz walks up and asks how I'm doing. Suddenly I burst into tears. "I just want to hold her!"

Pat looks over at him. "Can't we do something?" she asks. He looks down at me with pity.

"Alright," he says. Pat and another nurse help him remove the oxygen hood and rearrange the wires. Pat wraps Casey in a blanket and gently lays her in my arms while Dr. Fitz holds the oxygen tube up to her face. "Just for a few minutes," he says. As Pat grabs her Polaroid to snap a picture, Casey opens her eyes and looks up at me.

"Oh you're awake! How are you, precious? It's okay, Mommy's here. Don't be scared. Everything will be okay. Mommy loves you so much. I've waited so long for you," I tell her, stroking her cheek.

"Okay, Mrs. Novak, we need to put her back now," says Dr. Fitz.

"I'm sorry I can't hold you longer. Don't worry, Mommy's right here." They lift her from my arms and lay her back in the bassinet, quickly putting the oxygen hood back over her head.

"Do you feel better now?" he asks, smiling at me.

"Yes," I answer, smiling back. "Thank you."

~ ~ ~

When Casey's oxygen hood finally comes off, I spend my time between holding her in NICU and pumping breast milk in my room. Kathy and other long-distance friends and relatives call every day. Friends come every night, old and new, with arms full of gifts, and I share Miranda's scrapbook with them one by one.

Every morning Pat comes in, sometimes on her own, other times because I've called in a state of distress, and sits with me holding my hand as I cry. One of the nurses who took care of me after Miranda's delivery comes in. And Candy, who counseled us through our grief that awful week, comes too. I tell her how thankful I am she had been there with us, helping us, and taking pictures. After spending a year in a support group, I came to learn how blessed I had been. Some parents had no support in the hospital and left without memories, without pictures, without anything at all.

I ask where my favorite nurse, Carla—formerly known as Sergeant Carter—is and am disappointed when Pat tells me she moved away.

After five days, Casey is discharged. I was supposed to have gone home after four days, but Dr. Ross arranged it so I could stay an extra day until Casey was ready to come home with me. After my dad helps me dress her in a new sleeper, the nurse's aid wheels me down the hall, and I smile down at Casey trying not to think about the last time I was wheeled out of this hospital.

I'm greeted at home by a white stork sign in the front yard that reads: Cassandra Jane, 7 lbs. 8 oz., 5-12-97. I've waited so long for this baby, I want the whole world, or at least the residents of the Heritage Creek subdivision, to know she's finally arrived. In the backyard is our new tree, planted by the nursery workers coincidentally on the day Casey was born, and aptly nicknamed the "Casey tree."

That night, after I finish tucking Casey into her crib and softly kiss her forehead, I sit down in the rocking chair and watch her sleep. On her dresser next to the crib sits a stuffed bunny dressed in Miranda's hospital gown, cap, and ID bracelet. Above the crib, an angel hangs on the wall, a gift from Al's mom to watch over us after Miranda died. It seems fitting she should now watch over our new baby.

"Miranda, what do you think of your new baby sister?" I ask out loud. "Does she look like you? I think so too."

29

I'm so wrapped up with taking care of Casey, I don't have much time or energy to think about Miranda, until June 20th rolls around. Other than putting a candle in a cupcake and singing happy birthday to her, I haven't planned anything special like last year's impromptu beach outing. I spend most of the day wandering around the house, unable to focus on anything other than those painful moments when I held my stillborn baby and kissed her goodbye for the last time. Alex keeps asking why I'm crying. "Mommy misses your little sister Miranda." I get out Miranda's book to show Alex her baby sister's pictures again so she'll remember.

Beth calls around 5:00 p.m. "How are you doing?" she asks.

"Not so good. I thought the second year was supposed to be easier than the first year. This caught me off guard. I really miss her."

"I know. Yesterday was Joshua's birthday and it sucked. We're coming over tonight."

"Thanks Beth, I would really like that."

After putting their kids to bed, Beth and Heidi come over with a six-pack of beer and a chocolate pie. Brittany's birthday was two weeks ago, and Heidi is feeling the same emotional aftershocks that Beth and I are.

Wendy shows up with wine. "Hey, girlfriend, how are you?" she asks me.

"A lot better now that you're all here."

While my friends take turns holding Casey, I light three candles on the mantel in memory of our June babies.

"Hey Wendy, how's your new prayer group?" asks Beth.

"It's good, really good," says Wendy.

Wendy had learned about a prayer group at her church called Small Christian Faith Communities. She longed to have a deeper understanding of God, to somehow try to make sense of all that was happening in her life, and began attending the twice-monthly meetings.

Some of the women in Wendy's prayer group, older women who had been raised by traditional, conservative Christian families, held the belief that events in our lives, both good and bad, were God's will. Wendy often debated with these women that the loving God she knew would never purposely take the lives of her babies and cause her so much pain.

Although the belief system of each woman was different, their love for each other and dedication to God provided another form of support for Wendy. Wendy sometimes sat listening to the women talking about examples of how God sustains us, but often she shared her life and loss and asked for prayers. The women listened and prayed.

"How's Darlene doing?" I ask Beth and Heidi.

"I think she's doing okay," says Beth.

"Yeah, she started going back to support group meetings," says Heidi.

Darlene went back to the support group, this time with Larry in tow, and met a new friend who was a bank recruiter. The woman asked Darlene if she worked. Darlene told her yes, at The Baby's Room. "What? Are you insane, do you like hurting yourself? What are you doing?"

"Well, I needed to be around baby stuff."

"You are a glutton for punishment. You're never going to get any better if you don't get away from that stuff." She set up an interview at the bank and soon Darlene had a new job.

"Has anyone talked to Dawn?" asks Wendy.

"Yeah, has she put herself on bed rest yet?" I ask.

"Pretty much. I just took a meal over to her," says Beth.

Dawn's OB put in a cerclage, and although he didn't give her any restrictions, Dawn took it upon herself to become a couch potato. Andy supported Dawn's caution and at some point during the pregnancy, he wouldn't even let her push a shopping cart. She didn't lift anything; they didn't take long car rides; she did no cleaning. She wasn't doing much of anything, except concentrating on the growing life inside her. Neighbors and support group friends ensured that Dawn and Andy didn't starve by bringing dinner regularly. Everyone just wanted her to get through this.

So far, the pregnancy was uneventful, but Dawn was sensitive to things people were saying to her, like a neighbor who told Dawn everything was okay now that she was past the first trimester. Dawn had to tell her differently. When her doctor told her one day that everything was perfect, she scolded him saying, "Don't use that reference with me."

"Okay, I'd better make a note of that," he laughed.

As the months ticked by, there was little Dawn could do for her baby except to pray. Each prayer grew longer so that there was no question about what she was asking God for. "Please let my baby be born alive and healthy. Please let my baby be born alive and healthy and live a long life. Please let my baby be born alive and healthy and live a long, productive, healthy life." But Dawn knew from experience that sometimes even our most fervent prayers aren't answered the way we would hope.

"You know, Tracy is due right after Dawn," says Beth.

Tracy had made up her mind she would continue to go to support group meetings until her pregnancy started showing. Heidi and Beth were still going to meetings on occasion to support others, and both knew about Tracy's pregnancy, but she didn't share it at the group. She was there to work through her grief for Paul and didn't feel it would be fair to the newly bereaved parents to be talking about a new pregnancy.

For the first couple of months, Tracy went to the doctor every other week to check on the baby. She lived for the sound of the baby's beating heart—*thump thump, thump thump, thump thump.*

When she finally felt the first flutter deep within, she was elated, but then long intervals would go by without movement. Her anxiety began to build. She would sit at work in the hospital lab and think, *I wonder if this baby is alive or dead.* One day she went up to Labor and Delivery in desperation. "I'm having a really bad day. I haven't felt this baby move in a few days. I need to know this baby is still alive."

"Well you know with liability, we really can't," said one of the nurses. Tracy was a wreck and pleaded with them. The nurses gave in. "Okay, but we can't do this anymore." After a moment, Tracy heard the reassurance of her baby's heartbeat.

As her belly started growing, and she could feel the baby moving more regularly, she became more relaxed. She declined genetic testing; knowing about the possibility of birth defects didn't matter to them—they wanted the baby.

At twenty weeks, an ultrasound showed Tracy had placenta previa—the placenta was covering the cervix. Tracy went immediately to the library to get some books and learn all she could about the condition. Then she called Pat, crying, "I can't do this."

"Don't worry," Pat told her, reassuring her that if she started hemorrhaging, the medical staff should be able to stop it. Tracy was on pins and needles.

Wendy, Heidi, and Beth take turns passing Casey around, and the four of us laugh and cry, drink and eat pie, late into the night.

~ ~ ~

Later that summer, surrounded by family, Cassandra Jane is baptized in the church where, two years ago, we came together to say goodbye to Miranda. She's dressed in the booties, hat, and jacket that I suspect my grandmother had crocheted for Miranda. Finally, a baptism that I don't have to cry through. But I cry anyway.

~ ~ ~

In August, Dawn's water bag broke at thirty-eight weeks. At the hospital, her doctor's partner walked in—the same one who had delivered each of her triplets. *I can't do this. I can't go through this with him again,* she thought, remembering how he had run out of the room after each delivery. He surprised her by acknowledging that he remembered delivering the triplets, and that he was very sorry about what happened. He even remembered which delivery room she had been in.

At 8:00 a.m. Dawn's labor was induced with Pitocin. Soon, Dawn's labor came on strong; she felt out of control and pulled on the sheets. "It's hot in here," she complained.

"What do you need?" asked a nurse.

"I don't know what I need. I need to go pee! Just let me go pee, please will you just let me?" What she needed was someone to slap her. "I can't stand it, I need an epidural!" she yelled. Once they gave her the epidural, she was finally comfortable and could relax.

It was 10:00 in the morning. The doctor told them this was going to be an all-day affair; he was going home and would check back with them later. "Go get something to eat," she told Andy. "I need to rest." One of the residents came in an hour later to check on her.

"Um," she said, "you're going to have this baby right now. The baby's right here!"

"I thought that felt like a lot of pressure but, you know, my husband just went up to get a sandwich, and if he misses this baby, he's going to be really upset," Dawn said.

"And the doctor's not here," the resident reminded her.

"Well, I can wait as long as everything looks okay," said Dawn. "Can somebody go find my husband?" As the resident sent a medical student to the cafeteria, medical personnel filled the room. It was déjà vu as she flashed back to the triplets' delivery and she began to panic.

"Come over and look," a nurse told Andy as he rushed in. He hesitated. "Just come over here!"

"Yep, there's the hair," he told Dawn.

"We're trying to get the doctor back here," she said. "Are you okay? Just don't push!" Suddenly the doctor burst into the room wearing shorts and Dawn laughed as she suddenly thought of Kramer's wacky unexpected entrances into Jerry Seinfeld's apartment.

"What the heck is going on in here? Let me check you," he said, irritated. "Oh my God, you're going to deliver now!" He got prepped, took a deep breath, and turned to Dawn. With a calm voice he told her, "Okay, a couple of pushes and this is going to be over with." Within minutes, the baby slipped out. The cord was wrapped around its neck three times, but the baby was fine and let out a healthy cry.

They cut the cord and took the baby over to the warmer. The doctor congratulated them and told them he was so glad he could be involved with their happy outcome after everything they had been through.

"Excuse me," Dawn interrupted, "but can someone please tell me what the baby is?"

"Oh, you don't know?"

"No!"

"Well, it's a girl!"

Dawn had waited for a baby for so long; it had been three and a half years since the triplets died. Now, she sat in her hospital bed clutching Alyssa to her breast and crying. Heidi brought her the book *Love You Forever* and when Dawn read it to Alyssa, she cried even harder, tears of joy and sorrow. She loved this baby so much and was so happy to finally have her, but she also loved her firstborn children and realized now what she had missed with them. As she looked down at Alyssa, she wondered what it would have been like to hold three of them.

Two weeks after Dawn delivered, Tracy was induced. She was thirty-nine weeks, and although the placenta had torn away from the uterus slightly, it had moved up enough for a vaginal delivery.

She had begun to dilate, but her body wasn't ready to give the baby up yet and she and Jim walked the halls as labor dragged on. When contractions began to overtake her, she buzzed for the nurses from her bed, but nobody came. By the time they finally checked her, she was almost fully dilated; it was too late for an epidural. Instead, they brought her a huge red rubber labor ball nearly three feet in diameter and told her she could roll on top of it or hug it during contractions. Tracy wanted to shove that ball up the nurse's ass.

When it came time to push, the baby wouldn't come: it was stuck, like Paul had been, and the doctor used suction to pull the baby free.

The baby girl came out crying and the doctor immediately laid her on Tracy's chest. It was an awesome sound. Tracy was suddenly taken aback by the feeling of disappointment that the baby wasn't Paul. Yet, there was so much joy and relief to finally be holding a baby. "She's crying and she's beautiful and she looks just like her brother," Tracy cried to Jim.

Tracy was bleeding heavily and the nurse took the baby from her. "Tracy, I'm going to have to manually remove the placenta instead of waiting for it to deliver on its own," the doctor told her. After a few minutes he looked up at her. "The placenta has grown into the lining of the uterus. I'm going to have to scrape it out." The uterus, having been so stretched and thin, was at risk of being punctured. If this happened, Tracy would need an emergency hysterectomy. She was euphoric and didn't care what the doctor was going to have to do. All she could think about was her baby girl. At times during the past two years, Tracy thought she would never have a child of her own, not a live one anyway. Her uterus wasn't a concern right now. It had served its purpose and allowed Tracy to carry this child safely to full term. "I did the best I could," the doctor told her when he had finished. "But you might be passing chunks of tissue for awhile."

They called family to tell them baby Serena had been born, and everyone came with little girl outfits. It was a happy, wonderful day. How lucky she felt to have one that was breathing, a baby that she could take home.

Tracy bled so heavily her first week home, the doctor forbid her even to walk to the mailbox. She was content to lie around and nurse the baby. The weather was nice, and soon they walked every day.

Serena was a healthy, growing child, but still her mother worried about her. During the night, she would go into the baby's room and lay her hand on Serena's chest to make sure she was still breathing. When, at six weeks old, the baby slept through the night for the first time, Tracy woke up in a panic and rushed in to make sure the baby was alive.

Tracy joined a mom's group at the hospital for women who had just delivered babies. She met every week with her new friends, all of them younger than her. "We got pregnant on our honeymoon," said one. "The baby's only five months old and I'm pregnant again!" announced another. None of them had ever experienced a loss, and pregnancy for them was a happy, naïve, fun experience. Tracy shared with them what she had gone through and tried her best to educate them to be sensitive to other's struggles.

After three months, Tracy planned to return to work but struggled to find suitable daycare for Serena. She was afraid of losing her, too. She made appointments to visit homes that had openings, but felt that none of them were fit to leave a dog in. When Tracy finally found a woman she felt comfortable with, she began leaving Serena for only a few hours at a time and gradually worked up to a full day.

Tracy had finally fulfilled her dream of being the mother to a child she could care for, and she felt a completeness she had never known before. She thought she would be emotionally healed once she had another baby, but she wasn't entirely. She thought a new baby would fill that hole in her heart, but it didn't. She finally realized it was okay; the void Serena could not fill validated Paul's existence. That hole was Paul's special place.

~ ~ ~

In the fall, while Tracy, Dawn, and I stayed at home to nurse our babies, Beth, Heidi, Darlene, Wendy, Pat Vaci, and other local Share parents took a road trip to St. Louis for the National Share Conference and Walk to Remember. It was like going to a rock concert, except instead of a "We love you Bono" sign, they carried a banner with the names of their babies. Each of them had also brought a teddy bear wearing a baby-sized t-shirt with the names of their babies painted on the front.

Excitement buzzed about this year's keynote speaker Richard Paul Evans, author of *The Christmas Box,* the book Al had given me, about a parent's love and the loss of a child. Beth was especially excited. Although she had bought the book before she was pregnant with Josh, she didn't read it until after she had lost him. She loved it so much, she gave it to her sister to read on an airplane during an upcoming trip. When her sister landed, she called Beth.

"Beth, do you know where I am?"

"No," answered Beth.

"I'm in Salt Lake City."

It was the setting for *The Christmas Box* story. Her sister went to the cemetery where *The Christmas Box* angel statue now stands, laid white roses at the foot, took a picture, and brought it home for Beth. The gesture brought Beth closer to her sister who, not having any children of her own, had always struggled to understand Beth's grief.

At a workshop about men and grief, Beth got up to ask a question and was overcome by tears. An older man, who had lost his daughter many years before, consoled her. At the luncheon that afternoon, the man came over to Beth and introduced her to his son,

Richard Paul Evans. Beth started crying and told him how much his book had meant to her.

The overall message of the conference was clear: it was okay to still feel pain, hurt, resentment after one year, even after several years. One of the speakers struck a chord in Wendy as she talked about healing. "In your heart, go to where there is love." Michael, she thought. He was love. He was there, right in front of her all along. But she had been so grief-stricken and so focused on having another baby that she had neglected him. Sure, she had met his basic needs: food, clothing, bathing. But her mothering hadn't gone much beyond that. Where had the days gone? What had she been doing, and more importantly, what had Michael been doing? That night she wrote in her journal.

> *Dearest Michael,*
>
> *You were supposed to be David's big brother. You two were supposed to be a team. It is really difficult for me to give up that dream of brothers playing and getting into trouble. Taking you and David around to the grocery store, to the park, so many places, and being so proud of my boys, my little team. I wanted you to have a person to share your toys, your dreams, your frustrations about your parents…*
>
> *In my mind, I had so many plans for you both. When I see two little boys with their arms around each other, I weep for what could have been, not just for lost dreams, but for the gifted connection between brothers.*
>
> *Now, I pray for a connection between you and your father or your cousin or a friend (if we never have another baby). I'm working on making our relationship stronger. I want to be a good mother to you. You mean the world to me and I am so very, very fortunate to have you for my son.*
> *I love you,*
> *Mommy*

During a memorial service at the end of the conference, as she watched a family go up to get a rose after their daughter's name was called, Wendy was suddenly filled with the feeling that she would be blessed with another baby. It was like a light shining down on her. *This is going to happen. This will be okay,* she told herself once again. Shortly afterwards she found out she was pregnant.

Mark had absolutely not wanted to try for another one this time. But Wendy wouldn't give up. At six weeks, she heard the heartbeat. She cried, praised the Lord, and kissed her doctor. She went back at eight weeks and the heartbeat was gone. *You are a fool! What were you thinking?* she berated herself. She had to call Mark to meet her at the doctor's office. "It's bad news," she told him. He said nothing. *What did I do to deserve this?* she kept asking herself. Or was she asking God?

Wendy underwent another D & C to remove the child she had named Elizabeth, her fourth baby lost. It was December and she functioned on automatic pilot. She didn't go to the Christmas memorial service because she couldn't bear to put four angels on the tree. At home, she bought herself a new tree and lavishly decorated it with angels, ornaments, and ribbons of gold and sat in front of it every chance she could. She kept thinking about what age David would be—it was harder to keep track of the others.

"Mommy, do all babies die?" Michael asked his mom.

30

The sun streams in on a June morning as I sit on the floor watching one-year-old Casey stack blocks, the music of Kenny Loggins' *Return to Pooh Corner* playing softly in the background. Miranda's third birthday is approaching. Not a day has gone by during the past three years that I haven't thought of her at least for a fleeting moment. But every June always brings out remnants of emotions that have been deeply buried since the previous June. Journaling is something I've never done, but I'm compelled to pull out a notebook and put my thoughts down on paper.

Miranda, you would be three years old this month. When you died, I stopped taking things for granted—my life, my family, everything. But over the past three years, I've found myself slipping back into that pattern. Your daddy and I finally went out to see a movie and get a cup of coffee last night. But before this, I can't remember when we last took the time to have fun together, just the two of us. By the end of each day, we're exhausted. Come the weekend, there's an endless list of projects to do or errands to run. Tomorrow, I'll sit on the floor and play with Casey, I tell myself. "If I could just get this one last thing finished, then we'll do something fun,"

I promise Alex. I say these things every day with the false belief that there will always be another tomorrow. But I, of all people, should know there's no guarantee of that. When I find myself getting lost in a sea of busyness, I have to stop and remember that all I have is here and now. Would I know these truths, Miranda, if you hadn't left? I wonder.

Brittany's birthday has just passed, and Joshua's and Miranda's are next. I open the mail to find a birthday party invitation; this is no ordinary party.

WE'RE 3!!!! (sort of)
Joshua, Brittany & Miranda
(through our moms of course)
extend an invitation to you
for an afternoon of friends, food,
and remembrance.

What: A picnic to commemorate the birthdays of Joshua, June 19, 1995; Brittany, June 7, 1995; and Miranda, June 20, 1995

Who: You, your spouse, your kids, your friends, your priest, your shrink, your OB/Gyn and anyone else you want to bring

Where: Josh's place at Elm Lawn Cemetery

Time: 12:00 (noon, not midnight)

Bring a blanket or chairs and your own drinks. I'll bring the grub (that would be food, not grubs which are similar to slugs, which actually are already there).

I burst out laughing. *Only you, Beth!* In addition to Beth's wacky sense of humor, she has a gift for celebrating. When her dad died, she hunted down musician Ted Aliotta of Aliotta, Haynes, and

Jeremiah to come to the memorial service and sing their 1978 hit "Lake Shore Drive"; it had been her dad's favorite song.

The day of the picnic is beautiful, warm, and sunny. Heidi and Beth are kneeling on a blanket, spreading out food and drinks for everyone, while their little ones, Kaitlyn and Abigail, chase big brother David, eight, and big sister Madeline, five. Heidi is four months pregnant. She found out on April Fool's Day. At six weeks she went in for an ultrasound and they couldn't find the baby. One week later, they saw the baby, but after another week there was no change in the baby's growth, she was bleeding, and it looked like she was going to miscarry. At twelve weeks, the baby was still hanging in there, but cramping and bleeding was on and off again, and Heidi's fear of losing the baby grew. Heidi has a gut feeling she conceived twins and then miscarried one.

Tracy and Dawn are trying to keep their ten-month-olds, Serena and Alyssa, on the blanket with them, but the crawling babies are more interested in grass. Dawn is also pregnant and five months along. When she unexpectedly found herself pregnant again, Alyssa was only seven months old. They suddenly had a lot to consider, like putting in another cerclage and borrowing another crib. But most of all, she had a seven-month-old baby to lift and take care of. She worried about doing something wrong to endanger the new pregnancy, but she no longer has the luxury of spending eight months on bed rest and has remained active.

When Wendy arrives with four-and-a-half-year-old Michael, he jumps out of the car and heads for the big kids who have also been joined by my five-year-old Alex. One-year-old Casey, who's still mastering her ability to walk upright on two feet, is torn between sitting on the blanket with the babies or trying to keep up with the older kids.

I'm glad Wendy is here, knowing it must be hard for her to watch each of us with our babies and toddlers. After miscarrying Elizabeth last December, Wendy took matters into her own hands and started searching for answers to her questions. Each of Wendy's four losses seemed to be different, and she couldn't put the puzzle pieces together.

She read about immune response studies and learned about a blood panel—a series of tests run on her blood—that might be her only hope. Wendy consulted with a doctor downtown who took on cases other doctors wouldn't even attempt. The doctor's bulletin board was covered with baby pictures—evidence of her success—but she wasn't in Wendy's health insurance network. So Wendy went to see an endocrinologist in her network and asked him to do the blood panel. He told her it was expensive, about $700, and her insurance wouldn't cover it. After he read her chart, he said her problem was she "just had old eggs. Some people's eggs age faster. You'll just have to keep trying until you hit a good one." He also suggested she try an egg donor or undergo in-vitro fertilization. She was furious.

She paid to have the panel done, and when the results came back, she was looking at what might be the answer she had been looking for: an elevation in natural killer T cells. She consulted with the downtown doctor and learned these cells work against the baby, recognizing it as a foreign object, and then suppressing the hormones and processes the baby needs to survive. There was no way of knowing if these killer T cells were responsible for all or any of her babies' deaths, but at least now, if she became pregnant again, she would have a treatment plan.

Wendy turned once again to her journal.

May 8, 1998

I put away the baby bottle nipples today. As I took them from the shelf my eyes welled with tears. I felt myself resisting because these past days have been more peaceful and I couldn't afford another lost day. Well, the emotion of grief filled me and I let go of the tears! I may never have another baby. These past three years have been consumed with hope, joy, then disappointment, anger, depression, intense and dissi-

*pated grief all in the name of extending our family. I have to
let go. It's not mine to control anymore. I will pray for understanding and strength, and I will let go only with the help of
my dear Lord.*

Wendy had reached a point where she was determined to have
peace in her life no matter what the outcome was. But she hadn't given
up hope of having another baby. Now armed with information that
furthered her hope, she begged and pleaded with Mark to give her
another chance at motherhood.

Darlene is noticeably absent today. I know it has nothing to do
with the fact that she's the only one without a living child. She's told
us before: "It's okay for you all to have babies, because you lost babies,
but it's not okay for anyone else to have them." We laugh, but she's serious. There have been times, though, when we've gone on group out-
ings to parks, pools, and zoos, or hung out in a backyard, without
inviting Darlene. I get the feeling she's had some sort of falling out
with Beth and Heidi and they aren't talking. She's going through a
rough time. Beth tells us Darlene's younger, unmarried sister is
expecting a baby soon.

The kids kick balls and squirt each other with water guns from
behind headstones, and we laugh at how bizarre we must look to
people driving by.

Dawn and Beth are discussing cemetery plots. "Beth, you
picked such a beautiful site for Josh. Look at those rolling hills, trees,
and the pond," says Dawn. Then Beth tells Dawn how much the plot
cost, and Dawn laughs that her kids will stay right where they are.
When the subject turns to headstones, Beth says, "Okay, that's where
you made up the difference." Joshua's small stone laid flat in the ground
is modest compared to the triplet's towering three-foot stone that's as
large as the casket they were buried in.

"As big as the stone is," says Dawn, "the first engraver we talked
to told us quite bluntly that she wasn't going to be able to fit the

names, birth and death dates of three babies, plus the phrase Briefly in our arms, forever in our hearts. I walked out of there upset and determined to find someone who would help us. I found another engraver who came to my house with sketches and sat at our kitchen table with us. 'You can have whatever you want, honey. We'll make anything fit that you want,' she said, patting my hand. 'I know one day you're going to have kids here. My heart goes out to you. I'm so sorry this happened,' she said and hugged me on her way out. I was ready to invite her to Thanksgiving dinner!"

"For months, I was obsessed with how nice the cemetery plot looked," Dawn continues. "I watered the grass and trimmed around decorations with clippers. One time I forgot my clippers and got down on my hands and knees, trimming the entire plot with a pair of scissors. My hands were covered in blisters by the time I was finished. And over the years, my mom and I have bought enough cemetery holiday decorations to fill a storage unit. With all the plastic bags we've bought to keep them in, I should buy stock in Ziploc." Everyone laughs.

"Birthday" remembrance cards and flowers are handed out, and we finish our afternoon with a balloon release, each child sending love up to their brothers and sisters in heaven. We stare up into the blue sky until the very last balloon has disappeared from our sight.

~ ~ ~

That week, at my annual check-up with Dr. Ross, I give him the Anne Geddes baby photo book I bought for myself more than a year ago. With the birth of Casey, as well as my friends' babies, I've been reassured that pregnancy and childbirth can have happy endings. I no longer have need for it and know he'll appreciate it more. I'm thrilled when he smiles and tells me the famous baby photographer is his favorite.

Had I known Wendy had just discovered herself pregnant, I would have given the book to her.

31

It's November, and Beth and Heidi, who in addition to writing a newsletter for our local support group community, are now facilitating support group meetings with the assistance of a hospital chaplain, temporarily stepping in for Pat who's taking a break for a few months. I feel compelled to attend the meeting this month to offer help not only to grieving parents, but to Beth and Heidi as well.

"How's Jessica doing?" I ask Heidi after a hug.

"She's good. I think she's coming home soon."

Thirty-two weeks into her pregnancy, Heidi woke up early one morning and found herself bleeding. She called Beth to say she was driving herself to the hospital. "You're not driving yourself," Beth told her. "I'll be there in a few minutes." Scared to death she was losing the baby, Heidi grabbed a brown paper bag and began shoving things in: bras, a curling iron, a camera.

On the way to the hospital, Heidi yelled at Beth to keep going through the red lights. "Just go. Just get there!" She poked her belly every few minutes, convinced that the baby had died.

By the next morning, still contracting, she called everyone from the hospital to say she was delivering. The baby was coming and she was alive and Heidi didn't care how many weeks early she was. The birthing room filled quickly while the music of *The Christmas Box*

CD—based on the bestselling book—played in the background. Wendy, who was now four months pregnant, arrived to help. She and Beth sat alongside Heidi, Beth talking Heidi through contractions and Wendy using the Mr. Happy massager on Heidi's legs. Greg and Heidi's dad watched the Bears game, while Heidi's mom served as social coordinator asking if anyone needed a drink or a snack.

When it came time for the delivery, Heidi was told she could only have two people in the room. To her mother's dismay, she chose Greg, because he needed to have this healing experience, and Beth. After baby Jessica was delivered and rushed to the NICU, they popped open the champagne and Heidi got yelled at for mixing alcohol with medication.

Now, nearly three weeks later, Heidi is still wearing her hospital bracelet—she's at the hospital every day, nursing Jessica who's still in the NICU—and laughs that the new parents in the room tonight probably think she's escaped from the mental health unit upstairs.

Before the meeting starts, Beth and Heidi fill me in on Wendy's progress. In the summer, after Wendy found herself pregnant, she went straight to the successful downtown immunologist and began weekly blood draws, ultrasounds, and a monthly dose of immunoglobulin to suppress the killer T cells. She watched her new baby grow cell by cell. At the beginning of each appointment, she was haunted by memories of all those times when there was no longer a heartbeat. Her appointments caused her so much stress and anxiety that someone always went with her. When her mom wasn't able to go, Beth and Heidi, who both lived an hour away, took turns, one driving downtown with Wendy to her appointment, the other staying behind to watch all of the kids.

She treated each appointment as a girl's day out, always going for lunch afterwards, trying to make it fun again. In Wendy's case, it took more than two people to bring a baby into the world; it took an entire support system of family, friends, and medical specialists. And, it took a lot of money. But she was approaching age forty and needed to move on with her life. This would be her last baby, she had decided, and she was determined to enjoy every day as much as she could.

At ten weeks, she began seeing a perinatologist who also did ultrasounds and kept a close watch on her cervix. At her next visit, he noticed some changes and immediately put in a cerclage.

At sixteen weeks—the point she had gotten to when her bag broke and she lost David—the killer T cell level skyrocketed. Normally discontinued after the first trimester, the immunoglobulin treatments, they decided, would continue through the seventh month.

She loved being pregnant once the first trimester sickness was over. She even liked wearing maternity clothes. The best part was being able to let Michael put his hand on her and feel the baby move inside her. She clung to the hope of getting this baby through, but as each appointment approached, she reminded herself things could change at any moment. The baby was growing and developing, though, and things were going in the right direction.

They knew they were having a boy, and a small part of Wendy was sad because she would never have a daughter. She was glad she knew, though, because it gave her time to let go of her dream of having a girl. When Patrick arrived, she wanted it to be in full glory with no disappointment or regret.

The chaplain signals it's time to begin the meeting, and Heidi, Beth, and I take our seats. During the meeting, I feel a connection with a woman who's lost her full-term son to a cord accident. They've recently bought a larger house in anticipation of the new baby and are now in the midst of grieving and moving. After the meeting, I get her number and promise to call her later in the week.

Beth, Heidi, and I head for Omega after the meeting to have a bite to eat and catch up on our lives and the lives of the ones who aren't here.

Beth has started talking to Darlene again and tells us about Darlene's younger sister who gave birth to a daughter in August. When she got pregnant, everybody was happy for her—except Darlene, who was in a rage for months. She couldn't understand why her babies were taken away from her, while God would give a baby to somebody who had no husband and no money. The final straw was when she realized her sister was taking the baby stuff Darlene had asked her mother to store until the day she might need it again. "You're not getting this!" Darlene screamed at her sister, grabbing the Boppy pillow and ripping it to shreds.

Then she turned to her mother. "You talk about how this is your first grandchild, but it's not. This will not be your first grandchild. You were there, you saw the twins. You saw them before I saw them! She's using you. You're the one making the money and you're going to be taking care of her child while she goes on with her life as usual!"

"Darlene, this bothers me as much as it bothers you," said her mom. "But what am I supposed to do? I can't just kick her out, because the baby will suffer even more. I know you're upset that you don't have your babies. What you went through was the worst day of my life, and it's been hard to watch you go through this. I'm just trying to have a happy day with another baby."

Darlene looked at Larry. "Why doesn't this bother you?"

"I understand you're angry," said Larry, "but you're going to love this baby once she's born."

"I don't think so," said Darlene.

Her sister named the baby Kaitlyn Rose—the name Darlene had chosen in high school for the daughter she one day hoped to have—giving Darlene one more thing to be angry about. But Darlene's anger quickly dissipated when she saw her niece and learned she was born with a cleft palate. She took to Kaitlyn as if the baby were her own child, often taking care of her during the week, gently lifting her from the crib during naps just to hold her, spending weekends with her, and taking off work for the baby's corrective surgeries.

"Is Darlene trying to get pregnant?" I ask Beth.

"She's seeing a fertility specialist," she answers.

"I hope she can get pregnant again soon," I say. "She's been waiting so long."

"You know about Dawn, don't you?" Heidi asks me.

"No, what?"

"Last month, during a routine ultrasound at about thirty-four weeks, the doctor found something on the baby's brain. They told Dawn it might only be a cyst, but they can't be sure. They won't know anything until the baby is born and they do a biopsy. She's due any day now."

"She doesn't need this, after all she's been through," I say, shaking my head.

Later, I say goodbye to my friends and promise to see them at the Christmas memorial service next month.

~ ~ ~

Thanksgiving had just passed as Dawn neared her baby's due date. She and Andy were out shopping when contractions started coming every five minutes. "Why don't you call the doctor?" Andy urged. "I would rather go in today to have you checked than to wait until rush hour tomorrow morning," he reasoned.

"Well, I've got a bulb syringe, I've got a cord clamp, and I've got gloves," she answered. As a former labor and delivery nurse, she was prepared for anything.

He stared at her. "I'm not doing that!"

"But I've got it if we need it, just in case this is another fast delivery," she laughed.

Dawn's humor masked her terror of what they might learn once her baby was born and whether anything could be done about it.

"Stay near the shoulder of the road," Dawn told Andy on the drive to the hospital.

He looked over at her with panic. "Why?"

"No, I'm alright. Just in case." But she was becoming more and more uncomfortable. Every few minutes he looked over at her to make sure she wasn't delivering the baby onto the floor of the car.

When they got to the hospital, the staff was waiting for them with a wheelchair. She was dilated to two. "You're supposed to have extra people here because they think the baby has a cyst or something on the brain, and they want the baby checked out right away. The neonatologist is supposed to see the baby," she kept reminding the staff. "And I'm really uncomfortable. Why can't I have an epidural?" she pleaded.

Her doctor walked in and checked her cervix; by now she was at five. "Are you sure you really want the epidural?" he asked.

"Yes, please," she said through gritted teeth as she strained through a contraction.

"Okay, give it to her," he told a nurse.

Now comfortable and resting, Dawn was left alone. When they came in to check on her, they panicked. "Oh my God, this baby is right here!" Once again, everyone came scrambling from out of nowhere. Dawn was afraid to have this baby. She was afraid to find out what was wrong and wondered if the baby would be deformed.

Dawn pushed only once, and the baby slipped out so quickly the resident nearly dropped her. Kristen's cord was wrapped around her neck two times. But she looked perfect and was doing fine. Dawn held her new baby girl for only a moment before she was taken away to the NICU for evaluation.

It was late at night. Dawn felt numb. *I don't know if I want to hear this, I don't know if I can deal with this again. What's going to happen? Please tell me it's something that's going to go away on its own.*

Early the next morning, the doctors and nurses struggled to get Kristen to take medication to knock her out. She fought them with all her strength. Dawn was bawling. "I can't believe this is happening to me," she cried, preparing herself to lose another child. They got through the test and now it was a waiting game.

That night, as Andy left, he told Dawn he would be back at the hospital by 7 a.m. to meet with the doctor. "Don't worry about it," she told him, "If you're here, you're here. If not, I'll just let you know what he said." Andy couldn't believe what she was saying and wondered if the drugs hadn't worn off yet. Dawn was trying to convince herself this wasn't going to be a big deal; the doctor would tell her everything was fine.

The doctor came in the next morning and found Andy and Dawn waiting for him. "Your baby has a brain tumor," he told them. "We're going to do surgery in ten days."

Dawn lost it and began to cry uncontrollably. "I can't plan another funeral. I can't do this. This can't be happening to me!" she sobbed.

The doctor, unaware of her history, looked at her with surprise. "You don't understand," she cried. "We had triplets and we lost them. I've been through so much, I can't lose another baby!"

"Well," he told her, "if we don't take care of this now, she could end up with paralysis, or vision problems, or possibly she could die. We're going to let you take her home to get a little stronger and then bring her back in ten days. It's not something that needs to be done right away, but we can't let it go too long. We already have her scheduled." Dawn and Andy didn't have much choice in the matter.

They came home and had to call everyone to tell them the news. "We have a new baby girl, BUT she has a brain tumor." Dawn was beginning to agree with her friend who joked that Dawn was like bad-luck Schleprock, friend of Pebbles Flintstone and Bamm-Bamm Rubble, who walked around with a rain cloud over his head. She looked for blame in herself, just as she had with the triplets. She hadn't been as cautious with this pregnancy. Did she use a household cleaner that could have caused the tumor? Was it because she ate more junk food?

32

I feel as though the past three-and-a-half years have pointed to this moment. I've come full circle, from seeming wholeness, to devastation, to healing, growth, and finally back to wholeness. My support group friends, most of whom will be here today, have walked this path with me hand in hand. I am blessed and forever grateful for their lives, their laughter, their love.

Pat Vaci greets me at the door with a hug. I pick up a program and walk into the crowded room—the Christmas memorial service is about to start. Heidi and Beth are up front, lighting candles and arranging angel keepsakes. I take a seat next to Darlene, Wendy, and Tracy, reaching over to squeeze their hands. "Where's Dawn?" I whisper.

"She couldn't come. Kristen's brain surgery to remove the tumor is tomorrow."

Scanning the room, I see familiar faces from my early days of support group meetings, but so many are new. Beth told me five of the couples have had recent losses, in addition to sixteen "veteran" families here. I fantasize about the day when medical technology will become so advanced, there will be no need for pregnancy and infant loss support groups.

"Monica, are you ready?" Heidi nudges me and I'm pulled back to the crowded room full of bereaved parents. Taking a deep breath, I get up and walk to the podium. I take another breath, trying to keep my composure as I look into the eyes of friends and strangers who have found themselves on the same journey.

"Three and a half years ago, I lost my daughter Miranda. She was stillborn at full term. I don't have to tell you what I went through, because you all know. I didn't believe I would ever be happy again. Yes, I had a loving husband and a wonderful two-year-old daughter, but it wasn't enough. I wanted my baby girl back.

"Some of you might have been told by a well-meaning friend, 'At least you didn't know her.' Well, let me tell you my answer to that. I met her when I first heard her beating heart. Our relationship grew every time I felt a little thump that said, 'Hello Mommy.' I sympathized with her when the hiccups seemed to go on for hours. Like any proud mother, I watched her and my belly grow, little by little, day by day. I knew what her name would be and imagined her brown hair, hazel eyes, and long eyelashes.

"I knew the fun we'd have: the four of us walking hand in hand, one with Mom, one with Dad. 'Table for four, please'; ballet classes and Girl Scout meetings; catching frogs and fireflies; snuggling in for bedtime stories, one on my left, one on my right; baking cookies; daddy-daughter dances.

"I knew the adventures two siblings would have: playing make believe and hide-and-seek; building sand castles and snow forts. 'Wake up, wake up, Santa came!'; jumping in leaf piles and giggling under the covers; 'Mom, she took the last cookie!'; whispering secret messages through the heat registers.

"I knew the dreams I had: her first kiss, her first prom, her first heartbreak; football games and graduation, college dorms, wedding ceremony; her first baby, my grandchild. I know what could have been.

"Though we never brought her home, proudly displaying a stork sign in the front yard, I needed the whole world to know Miranda had been born. Though most of my family and friends never got to hold her close, or stroke her soft cheeks and dark hair, she had lived. Though

I would never get to rock her to sleep with a lullaby or nurse her at my breast, see her first steps, hear her first words, watch her grow up…I loved her as much as any parent loves a child. And there will always be a special, though empty, place in my life where she should have been.

"Danielle Steel wrote in her book *The Gift,* 'It's like some people just come through our lives to bring us something, a gift, a blessing, a lesson we need to learn, and that's why they're here. She taught you something, I'll bet…about love, and giving, and caring so much about someone…that was her gift to you. She taught you all that, and then she left. Maybe she just didn't need to stay longer than that. She gave you a gift, and then she was free to move on…she was a special soul…you'll have that gift forever.'

"This is the season of giving, and I'd like to share with you some gifts Miranda has given me.

"She taught me to pay attention to life. It wasn't until she left her earthly body that I realized how precious human life is and, as we're all too painfully aware, how short it can be. I may or may not have a future, and all I'm guaranteed of is right here, right now. So when I remember to, I slow down and try to deeply enjoy my favorite things: dancing with my daughters, listening to my husband play the guitar, watching the horses run across the field at the nearby stables, noticing the beauty and scent of each flower in my neighbor Alice's garden.

"Miranda gave me the gift of compassion, encouraging me to reach out to others. Before I lost her, I was in my own little world with little understanding of pain and suffering. I've learned that almost every person I come into contact with has a story to tell, and as I pass people on the street or in a hallway, I wonder what sort of pain might lie under their polite smiles. Now, when I'm given the blessed opportunity, I ask.

"Miranda taught me about gratitude. After focusing for so long on what I didn't have, I finally realized I already had so much to be grateful for: my health, a family, a warm house on a cold winter night, the sun shining, hearing the words 'I love you.' And I learned to appreciate the small things that add richness to our lives and make it worth living. A phone call from a friend just when you need it most. Laughing at something funny (my husband would say The Three Stooges). Springtime, with its smells of fresh earth, sounds of chirping birds, daffodils and snow crocus poking up from the ground. Someone to hold hands with. Good food cooked by someone other than me. Actually, any food cooked by someone other than me.

"After the death of his fourteen-year-old son, Rabbi Harold Kushner admitted that he would give up all the personal growth he had gained after losing his son if he could have his son back. I concur, and I suspect most of you would, too. Despite the growth Miranda's short life has inspired in me, I would give it all up just to hold my child in my arms and have her smile up at me.

"As I stand here and look into the faces of my dear friends, I'm reminded of how far we've traveled on this journey together, each having been to our own private hell and back. Not back to the way things always were; no, we're forever changed. But back to the light of day, to a different take on happiness, a new appreciation for life. For most of us, the bitter tears have faded into the background. For some of us, whose pain is still raw, the struggle goes on. But wherever we are today, and whatever happens tomorrow, we're here for each other.

"I long for Miranda when I look for her with my human eyes, but when I use my soul eyes, somehow I know her spirit is with me. I know, I must believe, she's safe, she feels my love, she urges me towards peace and joy, reminding me it was there all along, in my heart. Her life had purpose, and someday, when I'm with her again, I'll finally know why.

"I wonder what gifts your beloved babies brought for you."

After the memorial service concludes, I help Pat, Beth, and Heidi pack up candles and leftover keepsakes. Heidi tells us that last month, on the day they brought Jessica home from the hospital on a chilly November day, the pink rosebush she planted after Brittany Rose died—*Brittany's rosebush*—welcomed them home with a single pink rose blooming full and bright.

~ ~ ~

At home, I hang a special new memento on the Christmas tree. Specially commissioned by Heidi and Beth, the glass stocking ornament is engraved with these words:

Miranda
Amidst the joy and laughter, our thoughts will turn to you.
Christmas 1998

~ ~ ~

Two weeks later, my grandfather, Papa, dies. I drive to my grandparent's house in Indiana where family is gathering. When everyone leaves to make funeral arrangements, I stay behind in the quiet house, attempting to nurse Casey in Papa's rocking chair. My eight-month-old, who has never passed up a feeding, keeps turning her head up to look at the blank white ceiling, smiling profusely. I see nothing, but she knows something, or someone, is there. I remember her smiling like this at Papa while he lay in bed just weeks before. My sadness is temporarily lifted, and I smile up into seeming nothingness, wondering if Casey sees Miranda in the arms of the great grandfather who wept for her that June day on the steps of our church. I'll miss him terribly, but somehow know he isn't really dead or unreachable as I'd once believed he would be. He's merely left his ninety-one-year-old, cancer-ridden body behind.

A few days later, as I smile down on Papa lying in his casket and find myself, without any hesitation, running my fingertips along what little white hair he has left, I realize I no longer fear death as I once did: the idea of it, the experience of it, the body, cold and stiff. Yet, when my Grandpa died many years earlier, I remember the fear that enveloped me, the feeling that this was wrong, that death shouldn't happen.

The fears and ideas I held onto for so long had nothing to do with reality and had been taught to me by society, religion, media. It now seems the most natural of life's events, a returning home after a journey.

When my Aunt Betty, who had lost a stillborn son followed by a miscarriage, passed away suddenly, my mother received an intuitive message from her: "Tell everyone I'm alright. I'm with my babies."

As I look back on the death of my own child, I do so not with horror or fear, but with a gentle sorrow. And as I turn and look ahead, I do so with the hope and anticipation of a future reunion. Miranda has given me a divine perspective of the cycle of birth, life, death, afterlife.

33

After Dawn's baby's surgery in December of 1998, an MRI showed that part of the noncancerous tumor still remained inside Kristen's brain, and at four months old, Dawn and Andy took her in for a second surgery. "Here we go again. Will she live or will she die? Kids, don't move over," Dawn said looking up to the sky, "you're not getting another playmate," she told her children in heaven, determined to hold onto the ones she had.

Two years later, in July 2001, Dawn gave birth to another child, a son named Andrew. He quickly became the center of attention for big sisters Alyssa and Kristen, who were close enough in age and features to pass for twins. Most of Kristen's brain tumor had been removed, and her condition remained stable.

As the years went on, the angels on Dawn's mantel were moved over to make room for photos of her living children, but all throughout the house are still the reminders of three tiny babies born too soon.

~ ~ ~

In March of 1999, Wendy had made it to thirty-six weeks when the doctor removed her cerclage. She dilated to five and was immediately hospitalized. Four days later, the nurses took her down to the Triage area of the ER to induce labor; there were no delivery rooms available. Wendy told them no. After losing four babies, she had waited a long time for this one and wasn't about to deliver it alone in Triage without her support system.

Finally, she was moved into delivery, and with Mark, her mom, Beth, and Heidi finally at her side, labor was induced. Beth and Heidi, who now called themselves The Doulas, were Wendy's labor coaches. They figured they had earned it after all those months of babysitting and hauling Wendy back and forth to doctor's appointments.

Two hours later, she delivered a healthy son, Patrick. Wendy was awestruck by the sound of his cries, and she cried with him as they placed him on her chest. This journey of hers had been so incredibly long. This was her little baby boy, and this was it. They took Patrick home the next day, a happy complete family.

But she soon realized it wasn't the fairy tale ending she had hoped for. Mark went back to work, and Wendy was left to care for newborn Patrick and five-year-old Michael. Suddenly she felt alone, missing the people who had helped her through the past four years.

Patrick cried all the time and seemed to always be hungry, never satisfied no matter how often Wendy nursed him. Exhausted, she sat up every night crying while struggling to get Patrick to sleep. She had been told she was a prime candidate for clinical postpartum depression because of all the losses and fluctuations in hormones.

Television self-help programs gave their opinions about what she should be doing to be a good mom, and how to do things right, but in the end they just made her feel bad about her mothering ability. She forgot how to simply rely on her own instincts.

Voices in her head began telling her, '*You're a bad mom; you're a bad mom,*' over and over all day, every day. She wasn't doing anything wrong; things just weren't happening the way they were supposed to, the way she had envisioned all along. She was so tired and frazzled that at times she felt as if she could throw the baby across the room. It wasn't long before she began having thoughts of killing herself.

Her marriage was a mess and she began telling herself she didn't deserve anything, that the kids would be better off without her. One day she went into the garage, turned on the car and sat staring blankly. Three minutes went by before she turned it off. Two weeks later she went into the garage again, got into the car, turned it on and sat waiting, this time for five minutes.

At the order of a psychiatrist, Mark took Wendy to the hospital where she stayed for six days, scared and crying, before they were able to stabilize her. Beth took care of Patrick while Wendy was in the hospital. Beth and Heidi were the only two of our group who knew what Wendy was going through. She had been too ashamed to tell anyone else. Finally, she was sent home with medication and a follow-up plan. Wendy started seeing a behavior-oriented doctor who set goals for her and helped her get out of the "bad mom" mode she had convinced herself into.

Wendy eventually pulled herself out of the postpartum depression and began living the life she had always wanted with her two boys, Michael and Patrick, now best of buddies. As her healed heart looked back on her struggles, she made one final journal entry:

Some people say that self-help groups are simmering pots for self-pity and excuses to be victimized. I know and believe the opposite. I knew pain, understood it, struggled with it, at times succumbed to it and then blended with it. What can a person do if she or he doesn't recognize loss? Both the support group and prayer group became a conch shell for that pain—echoing, absorbing.

Losing a baby is like standing in the middle of life and not having life. It's much more than an empty vessel, which still has its outside structure, the contents gone. Yes, your baby has gone and psychologically the structure has crumbled to nothingness. You're so interconnected that the leaving of the baby is unfathomable. The baby has not abandoned you, and you cannot abandon the baby. You have to leave also. There are

*women who get through miscarriage without feeling this way
at all. I only understand how it is with me.*

~ ~ ~

After losing Andrew to miscarriage, Darlene's attitude about a
new pregnancy was, "If it happens, it happens."

It didn't happen.

In the fall of 1997, after coming home from the Share conference, Darlene consulted with an infertility specialist who
encouraged her to try consistently and methodically on her own
for one year. She watched her younger sister carry and deliver a
baby girl, while nothing happened for her. She began a regimen of
fertility treatments that took her through another year. In
November of 1999, Darlene finally found herself pregnant, and just
in time. The medication caused such severe mood swings, Larry
could hardly stand to be in the same room with her let alone have
sex with her.

She bled from weeks twelve to sixteen, every day thinking she
would lose this baby, too. At thirty weeks, she went into pre-term labor
and pleaded with her doctor to let labor take its course. "Right now
her heart is beating, please just let her be born." But he convinced her
to hang in for at least two more weeks to give the baby more time to
develop. She was given medication, put on bed rest, and the hospital
began remotely monitoring her contractions. Two weeks later, Darlene
pleaded her case again. "Can we please take her out now while she's
still alive?" But her doctor told her that even a thirty-two-week baby
might be compromised, and it would be in the baby's best interest to
stay in her mother's womb.

For nine weeks, while Darlene sat helpless on the couch, Larry
did everything: laundry, cooking, dishes, and housework, while
working and going to school.

At thirty-nine weeks, Darlene, now off the medication, went
into labor. While she waited for a wheelchair at the hospital, her water

broke. Larry was so nervous, he began laughing uncontrollably, which caused Darlene to laugh, and more fluid gushed out.

When Darlene got up to Labor and Delivery and realized she was having this baby now, she panicked. She hadn't been able to take a Lamaze class. Beth and Heidi—*The Doulas*—were both on vacation. "How am I going to get her out? I don't know how to do this!" The nurses reassured her it was their job to help; they knew what to do.

When the nurse did an internal exam, she looked blankly at Darlene. "I think it's her head, but it feels weird," she said.

"Oh no, don't tell me something is wrong, we had ultrasounds!" said Darlene. Another nurse came in and checked.

"No, that's not her head, it's her foot."

The doctor came in and checked her, his face suddenly dropping. "That's her cord, her cord is coming out. Lay flat, we have to get you to OR!" The prolapsed cord posed a dangerous threat to the baby's oxygen and, with it, her life. Darlene worried that she would feel the pain as they cut her open for the emergency c-section. The anesthesiologist, concerned with Darlene's recovery, and her doctor, worried about getting the baby out, fought back and forth about whether to give her an epidural or a spinal.

"I don't care, just get her out, just make sure she's alive!" screamed Darlene. Within two minutes, the baby girl was pulled from her mother's womb.

Geneva was born with a cleft lip and palate just like Darlene's niece, Kaitlyn. But Darlene didn't care; she was healthy and she was alive and Darlene knew all about cleft lips and palates.

Wanting another child, a sibling for Geneva, Darlene continued to struggle with infertility while keeping up with Geneva, a beautiful little blond, full of energy and life.

~ ~ ~

In the fall of 1998, Tracy's baby, Serena, was walking and talking, and Tracy and Jim tried for months to get pregnant again, wanting a sibling for their little girl. A radiology test confirmed what Tracy
had begun to suspect ever since the complications during Serena's
delivery: her uterine lining, a mass of scar tissue, wasn't intact enough
to carry another pregnancy. The doctor didn't have the heart to charge
Tracy for the test.

Tracy was frustrated and angry as she watched all of her friends
from Serena's playgroup having subsequent babies. She wasn't ready to
give up childbearing and found herself going through another grieving process. Tracy had grown up with two brothers and had never in
her dreams imagined she would have only one child. She tried talking
to Jim about adoption, but he wasn't interested.

The portraits on her bedroom wall—one of Paul, deceased,
one of Serena, living, painted by an artist from baby photos—would
be a constant reminder of the family that should have been. She was
so grateful to have that one child here to love, now a happy, healthy
little girl with her mother's brown hair, but Serena would be her only
living child, and Tracy knew something would always be missing in
her life.

Although the stuffed monkey never took another vacation
with Tracy and Jim, it remained a symbol of Paul and found a perma-
nent home on sister Serena's desk, leaving only at Christmastime to
resume his place of honor on top of the Christmas tree. The year Tracy
decided to do something different, decorating the top of the tree with
a big red bow, Serena brought the monkey downstairs and asked her
mom to please put it on the tree where it belonged.

~ ~ ~

Beth underwent surgery to reverse the tubal ligation she had
undergone after Abigail's delivery and began trying to conceive
again. Two years later, after undergoing six months of infertility treatments, she became pregnant. She miscarried at seven weeks. Beth let

go of the idea of another baby and kept busy with Madeline and Abigail, both blonds with big eyes and long, thick eyelashes, and now both in school.

~ ~ ~

Heidi's life quickly filled with carpooling David, Kaitlyn, and Jessica—one brunette, one redhead, and one blond—working in her pediatrician's office, and editing *Love Notes,* the local Share newsletter.

After calls for Heidi's and Beth's doula services tapered, they both enrolled in nursing school.

~ ~ ~

On a Monday in August of 1999, Dr. Ross delivered my *fourth* daughter, Anna, once again on his day off. Alex, Casey, and Anna became best of friends when they weren't busy being the worst of enemies. Through the years, Miranda has become ingrained in my children's hearts as if they've known her for an eternity: from Alex's kindergarten paper, "I feel sad when: Miranda died" complete with pencil drawing of a small baby in a box, to Casey's family drawings with four children, and Anna's stories shared with teachers and Girl Scout leaders about "my sister Miranda who died and lives in heaven."

Now when I'm asked how many children I have, I give my one and only answer: "I have four daughters. Three living, and one in spirit."

Although I haven't discovered with certainty the real meaning of Miranda's short life with us, I do know one thing for certain: Her coming and leaving has given my life new meaning, and I'm grateful for that.

~ ~ ~

September 2002

Smile!" shouts Beth's husband, Jeff, with his camera focused. Dawn, Beth, Heidi, Darlene, Tracy, Wendy, and I wrap our arms around each other and smile for a picture at our annual seven-family picnic at the park, seven years after those early support group days began. As the children play around us, and our husbands talk careers and sports, my six friends and I reminisce about our journey.

We started out like sorority sisters—the incoming freshman class—from scattered towns and different backgrounds, all drawn together, bound by this one thing. It was as if we had made a pact, somewhere in another time, to find each other in the midst of our tragedy, to climb out of it and grow through it, together. We became soul sisters. We supported each other, yet didn't realize we were doing it; it was simply a means of survival. How we looked forward to those monthly Share meetings, counting down the days until we could all be together again to share our recent ups and downs. Sometimes those nights went on forever. It didn't matter what we had to do the next day—this was our night and it was top priority. Our lives went on, but with an added dimension of wisdom and compassion.

I think most of us would agree that before our losses, we lived in somewhat of a dream world in which nothing as tragic as the loss of a baby could possibly happen to us. That naïveté gave way to a feeling of total vulnerability in the face of life's uncertainties. But as we journeyed together, and grew stronger, eventually coming out of the grief, we found a sense of peace in the knowing that if we could survive this, nothing could ever shake us completely from our foundations. What freedom there is in that knowing.

Although my six friends and I went in new directions and our time together has waned, our heart connections remain strong. Many of us, led by Heidi and a group of dedicated parents, were involved in the building of an angel garden at the hospital where Miranda was born and where our friendships were forged. It's a beautiful, tranquil place with water, flowers, trees, bricks engraved with names of little souls, and benches to sit and think, pray, and talk to our babies.

Often we run into each other at Share events such as memorial services and angel gardening days, or fundraisers like the annual luncheon or the Walk to Remember. Sometimes we pick up the phone to chat or e-mail each other for an impromptu rendezvous at the zoo or the pool; not often enough we meet for a girls' night out, sharing our lives and telling stories, like Heidi's story of the summer day that Brittany's magical pink rosebush had bloomed on June 7th— Brittany's "birthday."

We try to remember each other's babies on anniversary days, sending cards or flowers, or making phone calls. And, of course, every year we try to schedule our annual family picnic.

A friend who knows the story of the seven of us once expressed her amazement that our marriages had all survived given the stress we had been through following the deaths of our children. I told her I believed it was, in part, because we had the support group and we had each other during the darkest days of our lives.

Beth never did open the "Good Grief" store, but the name came to symbolize our group. Over the years, we had taken our grief and turned it into something good: courage, hope, friendship, and compassion for other bereaved parents who unexpectedly found themselves new members of our "club." And for the rest of my life, I will never be able to eat French toast (hold the beer) without smiling and thinking of my friends from *The Good Grief Club.*

"Say cheese!" shouts Beth. On the picnic table, squirming and scooting, smile our fifteen earthly children, while from somewhere close to our hearts smile our eighteen spirit babies.

34

July 2003, one year later...

On a summer morning, I sit alone at the kitchen table watching the last remaining drops of a heavy rain shower fall from the sky. My thoughts unexpectedly wander to that evening concert one warm July evening exactly eight years earlier when the feathery white puff I called a "flying fluff" floated around my hand. How unlikely the episode seemed, that I somehow believed my pleas for a sign from the heavens had been answered in the form of this small feathery ball, dancing around my outstretched hand like a playful puppy who never strays far from his master's side.

The memory comes and goes—why, I can't recall—but brings a smile to my face.

Shortly afterwards, as I walk down the driveway to let the kids in the van for the morning carpool, I'm stopped in my tracks by the sight of a flying fluff floating over my shoulder. It can't be. Everything is soaked from the rain. The air, still and heavy with humidity, hasn't been able to dry a thing, much less blow it off a tree into the air. Physically, this shouldn't be happening, yet it's unfolding before my eyes.

I begin to laugh. "Look girls, look at the flying fluff!" The kids stop and watch me with confusion and curiosity as I reach out my hand and gently scoop the flying fluff into my hand, watching it do its dance. A warm excitement, like the moment of a first kiss, pours through my heart.

I look up into the sky with a smile.

"Miranda?"

THE END

Epilogue

Through the years, the people who sought out our support group were as diverse as their circumstances. They were all parents with broken hearts, they all gave and received, and it didn't matter that they came from different backgrounds: a fourteen-year-old homeless girl who lost a full-term baby sat across the circle one night from a successful doctor who had lost twenty-two-week twins; a woman who, unable to have her own children, welcomed home an adopted infant only to lose her six months later; a single man grieved alone after the loss of his baby girl; isolated by distance, a grandmother mourned for her infant granddaughter who had died in another state. Like the well-known phrase, the playing field had certainly been leveled with the deaths of our babies.

Perhaps the stories that pain me the most are of the women who lost their babies many years earlier, at a time when support wasn't offered. Generations of women were told by husbands, mothers, doctors, and the rest of society to forget about their dead infants. Many weren't allowed to see or hold their babies. Funerals were often held without the mother; sometimes bodies were disposed of without a trace. These grieving mothers were led to believe that if they didn't think or talk about their babies, the pain would eventually fade away and life would return to normal. Kathy was one such woman.

On New Year's Day, 1971, Kathy gave birth to twin boys, Timothy and James. James, only three-and-a-half pounds, developed severe jaundice and four weeks later Kathy was told her son had a fatal liver defect. James never left the hospital, and on March 16th, died in his incubator while Kathy, her husband, and mother watched helplessly.

She never held him—she didn't know to ask—and after the funeral, the young mother was encouraged to forget and move on, often hearing, "But you still have your other son." She was so afraid of losing another child, she never became pregnant again—undergoing tubal sterilization to permanently prevent pregnancy—and her son grew up without a sibling. She and her husband grieved so differently, there was no support to help them through it, and within four years the marriage ended in divorce.

Now a young, single mother, Kathy grieved silently, overcome by depression every year during the holidays and the days leading up to the March anniversary of her son's death. For thirty years not a single day went by that Kathy didn't long for her son James, but the emotions remained buried in her heart—until the day her living son, Tim, and his wife Julie, after struggling four years to get pregnant, gave birth prematurely to triplet girls. One by one, Kathy watched each child take its last breath. The most tragic event in Kathy's past was now replaying in her son's life with the deaths of her three granddaughters, opening an old wound that had never healed and throwing her into deep depression that kept her confined to the couch for the next four months.

When Kathy began attending the support group with her son and daughter-in-law, the pain that had remained dormant for so many years came pouring out. And for the first time in her life, she was on a journey towards true healing.

I can't help but wonder how many women in our world carry old embers of grief in their hearts for children that should have been. Every son or daughter we bring into this world, whether it's the first or fifth, has a lifelong impact on us and our families. When a baby dies, we feel the absence of that child for the rest of our lives. Yet, we don't have to remain in grief. I believe our babies are whispering in our ears, *"Let go of the pain and be whole again. We're always with you."*

Resources for
Pregnancy and Infant Loss

If you are a bereaved parent, grandparent, sibling, family member, or friend, you are not alone. Help and support is readily available from caregivers and compassionate people who have walked the same path. Any one of the following organizations can help you on your healing journey by providing you with or leading you to one-on-one counseling, local support groups, online support groups, chat rooms, and message boards, newsletters, books, pamphlets, baby mementos, and memorial service resources. Some of these organizations also support families specifically through subsequent pregnancy, infertility, loss of multiples, or ending/continuing a pregnancy with a prenatal diagnosis of fatal birth defects.

If you are a caregiver at an institution that is lacking in its support services to bereaved parents, some of these organizations can provide training, education, and other resources and materials to help you better care for families following the loss of a baby through miscarriage, stillbirth, and infant death.

Share Pregnancy and Infant Loss Support, Inc.
National Share Office
St. Joseph Health Center
300 First Capitol Drive
St. Charles, MO 63301
Toll-free (800) 821-6819
(636) 947-6164 / Fax (636) 947-7486
www.nationalshareoffice.com
Nondenominational nonprofit organization offering support worldwide since 1977, serves those whose lives are touched by the tragic death of a baby through early pregnancy loss, stillbirth, or in the first few months of life. Extensive network of local support groups, online message boards and chat rooms, newsletter, information packet, resource catalog and more.

Alliance of Grandparents, A Support in Tragedy (AGAST)

P. O. Box 271386
Salt Lake City, UT 84127
International Coordinator Toll-Free (800) 793-7437
Executive Director Toll-Free (888) 774-7437
www.agast.org
An international all-volunteer organization dedicated to helping grandparents through the trauma, stress, and grief after the loss of a grandchild. AGAST supports grieving grandparents with information packets, personal contact, remembrance cards, and newsletter.

Bereaved Parents of the USA

National Office
P.O. Box 95
Park Forest, IL 60466
(708) 748-7866
www.bereavedparentsusa.org
Offers support, understanding, encouragement and hope to bereaved parents, siblings and grandparents, and educates families about the grief process pertaining to the death of a child at any age and from any cause through local support group chapters, a national newsletter, brochures and other resources, and an annual gathering.

Bereavement Services

Gundersen Lutheran Medical Foundation
1900 South Avenue, ALEX
La Crosse, WI 54601
Toll-free (800) 362-9567 ext. 54747
(608) 775-4747 / Fax (608) 775-5137
www.bereavementservices.org
Provides clinically-based professional training for caregivers, publishes newsletter, and offers catalog for resources and gifts with quantity pricing.

Center for Loss in Multiple Birth (CLIMB), Inc.
P.O. Box 91377
Anchorage, AK 99509
(907) 222-5321
www.climb-support.org
Nonprofit organization by and for parents who have experienced the death of one or more, both, or all, of their twins or higher multiples during pregnancy, at birth, in infancy or childhood. Offers newsletter and parent network.

Centering Corporation
7230 Maple Street
Omaha, NE 68134
Toll-free (866) 218-0101
www.centeringcorp.com
Nonprofit organization founded in 1977 dedicated to providing education and resources for the bereaved through extensive catalog of books, videos/DVDs, CDs, cards and more. Offers education, workshops, and online forum. Publisher of Grief Digest.

The Compassionate Friends, Inc.
P. O. Box 3696
Oak Brook, IL 60522
Toll-free (877) 969-0010
(630) 990-0010 / Fax (630) 990-0246
www.compassionatefriends.org
Since 1969, this nonprofit assists families toward the positive resolution of grief following the death of a child of any age and provides information to help others be supportive. Offers local and online support groups, magazine, and numerous brochures written exclusively by bereaved parents, grandparents, or siblings.

Compassion Books, Inc.
7036 State Hwy 80 South
Burnsville, NC 28714
Toll-free (800) 970-4220
(828) 675-5909 / Fax (828) 675-9687
www.compassionbooks.com
Resource catalog with more than 400 books, videos, and audios to help children and adults through serious illness, death and dying, grief, bereavement, and losses of all kinds including pregnancy and infant loss.

First Candle/SIDS Alliance
1314 Bedford Avenue, Suite 210
Baltimore, MD 21208
Toll-free (800) 221-7437
www.firstcandle.org
A national nonprofit health organization uniting parents, caregivers and researchers with government, business and community service groups to advance infant health and survival. Offers online resources, grief packets, referrals to local support groups, conferences, and crisis phone line for parents whose baby has died during pregnancy or after birth.

Grief Watch – Perinatal Loss
2116 NE 18th Avenue
Portland, OR 97212
(503) 284-7426 / Fax (503) 282-8985
www.griefwatch.com
Offers spiritual, emotional and other support to persons who are grieving. Grief Watch and its companion program, Perinatal Loss, publish books, videotapes, audiotapes and other helpful resources aimed at persons who have suffered loss. Publisher of Tear Soup, A Recipe for Healing After Loss.

Hannah's Prayer Ministries
P.O. Box 3321
Borger, TX 79008
Voice Mail / Fax (336) 848-1552
www.hannah.org
Provides Christian-based volunteer support and encouragement to couples around the world who are struggling with the pain of infertility, pregnancy loss, early infant death, and adoption loss.

A Heartbreaking Choice
www.aheartbreakingchoice.com
For parents who choose to interrupt their pregnancies after poor prognosis from prenatal diagnosis. Website provides articles, stories, online discussion boards, and resource listings/links.

M.I.S.S. Foundation
P.O. Box 5333
Peoria, AZ 85385
Toll-free (888) 455-MISS (6477)
(623) 979-1000 / Fax (623) 979-1001
www.missfoundation.org
Nonprofit, volunteer-based organization providing crisis support and long term aid to families after the death of baby or child from any cause. Network of local support groups, online live chat and message board, newsletter, information and resources, workshops and speakers.

Mommies Enduring Neonatal Death (M.E.N.D.)

P.O. Box 1007
Coppell, TX 75019
972-506-9000
www.mend.org
A Christian nonprofit organization whose purpose is to reach out to those who have lost a child due to miscarriage, stillbirth or early infant death and offer a way to share experiences and information through support groups, newsletter, ceremonies, and website.

A Place to Remember

1885 University Avenue, Suite 110
St. Paul, MN 55104
Toll-free (800) 631-0973
(651) 645-7045 / Fax (651) 645-4780
www.aplacetoremember.com
Provides uplifting support materials and resources for those who have been touched by a crisis in pregnancy or the death of a baby.

Pregnancy Loss and Infant Death Alliance (PLIDA)

P.O. Box 658
Parker, CO 80134
Toll-free (888) 546-2828, then press 3
www.plida.org
A collective community of parents and health care professionals, PLIDA's goal is to provide a formal network and a unified national presence to increase awareness and education on the emotional experiences and needs of bereaved families following the death of a baby during pregnancy, birth, or infancy. PLIDA advocates for the provision of supportive care to parents by providing support, education, and networking opportunities to the professionals who work with bereaved families.

Recommended Books

There are many wonderful books available from the organizations listed previously. The following is my own personal list of books that helped me heal along the way.

Angelic Presence: Short Stories of Solace and Hope After the Loss of a Baby
Cathi Lammert and Sue Friedeck (Evans Publishing, 1998)

A Silent Sorrow: Pregnancy Loss – Guidance and Support for You and Your Family
Ingrid Kohn, Perry-Lynn Moffitt, Isabelle A. Wilkins, MD (Brunner-Routledge, 2000, 2nd edition)

Dear Cheyenne: A Journey into Grief
Joanne Cacciatore (MISS Foundation, 2002, 5th edition)

Dear Parents: Letters to Bereaved Parents
Joy Johnson (Centering Corp., 1989)

Embraced by the Light
Betty J. Eadie (Gold Leaf Press, 1992)

Empty Cradle, Broken Heart: Surviving the Death of Your Baby
Deborah L. Davis (Fulcrum Publishing, 2004, 2nd edition)

An Empty Cradle, a Full Heart: Reflections for Mothers and Fathers After Miscarriage, Stillbirth, or Infant Death
Christine Lafser (Loyola Press, 1998)

Hannah's Gift: Lessons From a Life Fully Lived
Maria Housden (Bantam, 2003)

Life Touches Life: A Mother's Story of Stillbirth and Healing
Lorraine Ash (NewSage Press, 2004)

Spirit Babies: How to Communicate With the Child You're Meant to Have
Walter Makichen (Delta, 2005)

The Christmas Box
Richard Paul Evans (Simon & Schuster, 1995)

Waiting With Gabriel: A Story of Cherishing a Baby's Brief Life
Amy Kuebelbeck (Loyola Press, 2003)

When Hello Means Goodbye
Paul Kirk, MD and Pat Schwiebert, RN (Perinatal Loss, 1993, 2nd edition)

If you want to go back and reread something, here's where you can find it:

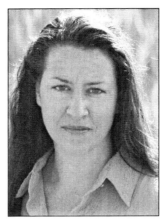

©Kelly Axtolis

MONICA NOVAK grew up in northwest Indiana and graduated from Purdue University with a degree in Business Management. Following the stillbirth of her daughter Miranda in 1995, she was moved by spirit to write the story of her journey with the women she befriended at a support group for pregnancy and infant loss, a bond that led them from a place of grieving to a new life of hope, healing, and happiness.

Monica shares her story with local and national audiences, and has supported bereaved mothers and fathers one-on-one. Her mission is to bring comfort and hope to bereaved parents worldwide and to educate and promote awareness and compassion to the physicians, nurses, clergy, counselors, family, and friends of every mother or father who has or ever will be told that their baby has no heartbeat or that nothing more can be done.

The full-time mother of three daughters, Monica lives in the Chicago area with her husband, children, and a rat terrier named Sami—short for Samantha.

For more information or to contact the author, please visit www.TheGoodGriefClub.com, or write to:

Monica Novak
P.O. Box 1035
Bolingbrook, IL 60440